CHILDREN AND AIDS

Global Health

Series Editor: Nana K. Poku,
Health Economics and AIDS Research Division (HEARD), South Africa

The benefits of globalization are potentially enormous, as a result of the increased sharing of ideas, cultures, life-saving technologies and efficient production processes. Yet globalization is under trial, partly because these benefits are not yet reaching hundreds of millions of the world's poor and partly because globalization has introduced new kinds of international problems and conflicts. Turmoil in one part of the world now spreads rapidly to others, through terrorism, armed conflict, environmental degradation or disease.

This timely series provides a robust and multi-disciplinary assessment of the asymmetrical nature of globalization. Books in the series encompass a variety of areas, including global health and the politics of governance, poverty and insecurity, gender and health and the implications of global pandemics.

Also in the series

The Politics of Surveillance and Response to Disease Outbreaks
The New Frontier for States and Non-state Actors
Edited by Sara E. Davies and Jeremy R. Youde
ISBN 978 1 4094 6718 2

HIV/AIDS and the South African State
Sovereignty and the Responsibility to Respond
Annamarie Bindenagel Šehović
ISBN 978 1 4724 2337 5

Living with HIV and Dying with AIDS
Diversity, Inequality and Human Rights in the Global Pandemic
Lesley Doyal with Len Doyal
ISBN 978 1 4094 3110 7

Informal Norms in Global Governance
Human Rights, Intellectual Property Rules and Access to Medicines
Wolfgang Hein and Suerie Moon
ISBN 978 1 4094 2633 2

Children and AIDS

Sub-Saharan Africa

Edited by

MARGARET LOMBE
Boston College Graduate School of Social Work, USA

ALEX OCHUMBO
Ethiopian Catholic University of St. Thomas Aquinas (ECUSTA), Ethiopia

Routledge
Taylor & Francis Group
LONDON AND NEW YORK

First published 2016 by Ashgate Publishing

Published 2016 by Routledge
2 Park Square, Milton Park, Abingdon, Oxon OX14 4RN
711 Third Avenue, New York, NY 10017, USA

Routledge is an imprint of the Taylor & Francis Group, an informa business

British Library Cataloguing in Publication Data
A catalogue record for this book is available from the British Library

The Library of Congress has cataloged the printed edition as follows:
Lombe, Margaret.
Children and AIDS : Sub-Saharan Africa / by Margaret Lombe and Alex Ochumbo.
pages cm. -- (Global health)
Includes bibliographical references and index.
ISBN 978-0-7546-7781-9 (hardback)
1. AIDS (Disease)--Africa, Sub-Saharan. 2. Child welfare--Africa, Sub-Saharan. 3. Children--Health and hygiene--Africa, Sub-Saharan. 4. Children--Social conditions--Africa, Sub-Saharan. I. Ochumbo, Alex. II. Title.
RA643.86.A357L66 2015
362.19697'9200967--dc23

2015010325

ISBN 9780754677819 (hbk)

Contents

List of Figures

List of Tables

Notes on Contributors

A unique characteristic of this book is the multidisciplinary perspectives that the contributing authors bring to this work. Contributing authors come from a range of academic disciplines and fields of practice. This diverse perspective is essential to a book of this nature. The issue of vulnerability, especially among orphaned children, reveals an intersection of a number of factors such as poverty, lack of access to education and healthcare services, social support, and how these interact to inhibit life chances for vulnerable children and their communities.

Margaret Lombe (PhD) is an assistant professor at the Boston College Graduate School of Social Work. She is also a faculty associate at the Center for Social Development at Washington University. Her area of expertise is in international social development with an emphasis on social inclusion/exclusion and capacity building. Margaret has provided consultation to the United Nations and has participated in a number of Experts Group Meetings (EGM), working with the UN to develop tools to assess inclusion/exclusion. She has published book chapters and a number of articles on the issue of social inclusion and AIDS; and has presented papers at both local and international conferences in this field. Her recent work has appeared in refereed journals including: *Journal of Human Behaviour in the Social Environment*, *Social Work Research*, *Journal of Community Practice*, and the *Journal of Sociology and Social Welfare*.

Protus Lumiti is Chief Manager of Nyumbani Children's Home, which is under the Children of God Relief Institute as a registered charitable organization in Kenya, USA, UK, Italy, Ireland and Spain. The home was founded by Father Angelo D'Agostino SJ.MD in 1992. The home supports children who are HIV positive in a residential environment and is situated in Karen, Nairobi. Protus has a Bachelor's degree in Philosophy from Urbanian University and a Bachelor of Arts from Catholic University of Eastern Africa. He earned his MBA from Kenyatta University. He is currently a third-year PhD candidate at Jomo Kenyatta University of Agriculture and Technology. He is a member of the Institute of Human Resource Management, associate member of Kenya Institute of Management and a founder member of Flomic Institute of Business Management. He is a member of Rotary International. Some of his unpublished research includes "The Impact of Constituency Development Fund in Kenya" (2008) and "Children and their Rights in Kenya" (2000).

Theresa Lungu was born and raised in Luanshya, Zambia and is the founder of Books for Zambia (www.Booksforzambia.com). A graduate of Boston College and recipient of the Dean's Award for Creative Writing, Theresa is also the author of the novels *Twilight in the Morning* and *Torment of an Angel.* She currently resides in Massachusetts and is an employee and student of Harvard University.

Harriet Mabikke (MSW) graduated from Uganda's Makerere University and Boston College's Graduate School of Social Work. Her area of interest is global practice, poverty, and vulnerable children. A native of Uganda, Harriet has worked with women in rural Uganda around issues of poverty reduction, and with orphaned and vulnerable children in Zambia. Harriet is President of Hope Networks International (HNI).

Lyndsey McMahan (BA, MSW) has experience working domestically in both child welfare and immigration related to asylum seekers. Her international work includes: two years as a Peace Corps volunteer in Mporokoso, Zambia, working with rural communities regarding safe health practices; community service activities in Mexico and Turkey; and project development and implementation including evaluation data analysis for HelpAge International in Cambodia. Lyndsey strongly believes in the social work Code of Ethics which promotes service, social justice, integrity, cultural competence, and the worth of human relationships—these are values that complement Lyndsey's goal of working in a field that promotes the understanding that every human life has a story and an inherent dignity that must be heard and upheld.

Tapologo Maundeni (PhD) is an associate professor in the Department of Social Work, University of Botswana. Tapologo has a PhD in Social Work from the University of Glasgow in Scotland. She has extensive leadership skills which she acquired through carrying out various assignments both locally and internationally. She has led numerous projects successfully and conducted several consultancies for international and national organizations such as UNESCO, DFID, and the Ministry of Health in the areas of children's rights, HIV and AIDS, and Social Safety Nets for People Living with Disabilities as well as Gender based Violence. Tapologo has also been active in community organizations throughout Botswana and the southern region of Africa that focus on child and family welfare issues, such as the National Children's Council, the Reference Committee that reviewed the Botswana Children's Act, the National Pre-school Development Committee, the sub-committee that drafted the child protection section of the National Plan of Action (NPA) for the children of Botswana, and the Department of Social Services' Committee that prepares for the annual commemorations of the International Day of the Family. Her areas of expertise are children's rights, gender, human rights, child and family welfare, and HIV and AIDS. She has published extensively on these areas. Her most recent publications include HIV/AIDS, Vulnerable Groups, Human Rights and Development in Botswana.

Mosidi Tseleng Cynthia Mokotedi (RN, MSN), has been a lecturer at the School of Nursing, University of Botswana, and Gaborone since 2008. She holds a BEd degree in Nursing from the University of Botswana and a MSc (Nursing) from the University of Technology in Sydney Australia. Mokotedi has worked at Mahalapye hospital as a midwife and lecturer at the Institute of Health sciences. At the University of Botswana, she has served on various departmental committees, faculty and university wide committees. She is a member of Africa Honor Society Chapter of Sigma Theta Tau International and of The Organization for Social Science Research in Eastern and Southern Africa; Botswana Chapter. Mokotedi is also a member of the Nurses Association of Botswana. She was an Internal Examiner for the Institute of Health sciences for three years. One of her publications covers the "Development and Evaluation of an interdisciplinary Palliative Care workshop in Botswana" and her ongoing research support includes: Challenges faced by parents with haemophilic children in Botswana and departmental study on maternal mortality in Botswana.

Chiedza Mufunde (MSW) currently works on research and policy development with "A World at School"—a global education campaign mobilizing various public and private institutions and partners on finishing the education goal of Millennium Development Goals. She is passionate about women's education and reproductive rights with an interest in policy and research. Her work with the Campaign for Female Education (CAMFED) in Zimbabwe inspired her passion for education and the importance of investing in women to fight poverty. She has interned with the Institute of Women and Ethnic Studies in New Orleans, the New England Alliance for Children's Health in Boston, MA, and Save the Children in Washington, DC, working on issues affecting children in health and education. She holds a BA Hons in Psychology from Mount Holyoke College in Massachusetts, and a Master's degree in Social Work with a focus on global practice and policy from Boston College School of Social Work.

Chrisann Newransky (PhD) is an assistant professor in the School of Social Work at Adelphi University in New York. Her background is in social policy and her current area of research focuses on the social determinants of health disparities and social exclusion/inclusion. Previously, she studied the capacity of self-help microcredit programs to enhance the health and welfare of women and children in sub-Saharan Africa and India. Chrisann has been a board member for Empower Dalit Women of Nepal (EDWON), a human rights organization for "untouchable" women. Prior to her graduate studies, she spent eight years working overseas for Habitat for Humanity International in the Philippines and for the local government in Japan. Chrisann earned her PhD and MSW from the Graduate School of Social Work at Boston College and also holds an MA in Sustainable International Development from Brandeis University.

Alex Ochumbo (PhD) is Vice President for Capacity Building and Research at the Ethiopian Catholic University of St. Thomas Aquinas (ECUSTA). He is also a member of the CORE Team that has been mandated by the Owners to implement the day-to-day activities and policies of the university. Prior to joining ECUSTA he worked for the Children of God Institute (COGRI), Nairobi, Kenya. His work involved counseling and offering spiritual guidance to children affected by HIV/AIDS. His main interest is in the area of sustainability of programs to assist HIV/AIDS children and orphans in sub-Saharan Africa. His area of expertise is in management, with an emphasis on international human resources management. Alex has worked at the administrative level with Jesuit Refugee Services and other organizations assisting refugees.

Ogar Rapinyana (RN, MSN) is a lecturer at the School of Nursing, University of Botswana, Gaborone. Ogar is a registered nurse midwife. She obtained her BSc degree at the University of Botswana in 1995 and her MSc degree in Midwifery at the University of Witwatersrand, Johannesburg, South Africa. She worked as an employee of the Botswana government for 20 years as a staff nurse and midwife at various clinics and hospitals. From 1995 to 1997 she held positions as: Assistant Lecturer, Lecturer, Senior Lecturer and lastly Coordinator of the Midwifery program at Institute of Health Sciences, Francistown, Botswana. She was a member of the Taskforce that reviewed the Midwifery Curriculum and Integrated the HIV and AIDS into the Midwifery Curriculum for the HIV programs at the workshop held in New Jersey, United States, in 2005. She has researched and presented conference papers in the area of Midwifery and HIV and AIDS. Ogar also served as an internal examiner for the Master of Nursing student research projects. She served as a representative of the School of Nursing at the Nurses Association of Botswana and as a board member of the Botswana Nursing Council. She is a member of Tau Lambda at Large Chapter of STTI and East, Central and Southern Africa College of Nursing for Africa ECSACON.

Naomi Seboni (RN, RM, PhD) is a senior lecturer in the School of Nursing, University of Botswana, Gaborone. Naomi is a registered nurse-midwife. She obtained her basic degree in Nursing at the University of Botswana and Swaziland in 1981, her Master's degree at Teachers College, Columbia University in New York, and her PhD at the University of California, San Francisco, in 1993. For her Master's degree, she specialized in adult health, and later focused on young adults (adolescent health and development) at doctoral level. Her PhD thesis focused on teenage girls' sexuality and sexual risk-taking behaviors. She worked as an employee of the University of Botswana (UB) for 29 years. She is the former Head of the School of Nursing and the Director of the WHO Collaborating Centre for Nursing and Midwifery Development at the UB, where she served in various Task Groups for WHO Africa Region and headquarters on issues pertaining to the development of nursing and midwifery. She has served as a consultant for the Ministry of Education, UNICEF and PATH in the area of adolescent sexuality and sexual behaviors. She has also researched and published in the area of adolescent health and sexuality, and adolescents living with HIV and AIDS amongst others. Naomi has provided leadership through her professional and community service to NGOs providing care to adolescents. She served as President for the Botswana Family Welfare Association, an affiliate of the International Planned Parenthood Federation (IPPF), and is currently a member of the African Regional Governing Council as well as the International Governing Council of IPPF.

Aakanksha Sinha (MSW) is a doctoral student at the Graduate School of Social Work, Boston College. Her main research interest is on issues concerning the wellbeing of orphan children, with a focus on community development and human rights. She also focuses on access to basic needs for low-income children and families in the global south. Presently, she is involved in research endeavors in the United States, as well as countries in the global south, that focus on protection and overall development of orphan children, through innovative projects such as cash transfers, community-based care, intergenerational community care, and others. She is also involved in research on food security and disabilities issues and how they impact the overall wellbeing and quality of life of communities in the United States and globally.

Nicholas Syano is a program manager at Children of God Relief Institute administering all the activities of Nyumbani Village and the community based programs. Nyumbani Village in Kitui, Kenya is a home for HIV/AIDS orphans and their grandparents living in conditions that make it possible for them to attend school, have accommodation and food. The grandparents grant them the parental guidance that they need while Nicholas is currently a PhD candidate of Dry Land Resource Management, Nairobi University and the chairperson of Dryland Natural Resources Centre (DNRC). He has a Bachelor of Science degree from Maseno University in Kenya and a Master of Science degree in Natural Resources Management from the University of Wisconsin, USA where he was the Kenyan In-Country Coordinator of Global Environmental Management Education Center (GEM). He was also the Center Manager of Kenya Institute of Organic Framing (KIOF), Kenya.

We dedicate this book to the African child and every child upon whom the label of vulnerability has been attached by those with the mandate to love, nurture and safeguard. We look into your eyes, we see capacity to dream and realize your potentiality. We salute you African child.

Preface and Acknowledgments

Many people and experiences inspired this book. It reflects our journey as we grapple with the challenge of growing vulnerability among children in sub-Saharan Africa. A major source of influence is our parents through whose eyes we learned to look at a child with reverence. We learned to believe in the virtue of *convivencia*; that you and I belong to the greater whole and that the child is the center.

Another source of inspiration are students at the Boston College Graduate School of Social Work, in the Global Practice field of study, who through the years have pushed us to question the universality of human rights. For years, together, we have wrestled with injustice but stand strong enough to dream of a world in which every man, woman and child, regardless of "isms," has validation. Together, we have learned to take steps toward that ideal—we believe that a just world in which children are valued is possible.

Colleagues in the field of social work have greatly influenced this work by providing a platform upon which to wrestle with challenging issues of this nature. Dean Alberto Godenzi deserves special mention for providing an environment that understands the intersection between human rights, health and social justice. We are indebted to Michael Sherraden for pushing us to look at the "why not?" and Kevin Mahoney for graciously listening as we tried to make sense of the rights of the child within the African context.

Perhaps, the most significant inspiration of all has been the children classified as "vulnerable" whom we have interacted with in our own families, communities and as researchers. We have looked into their eyes, held their hands, played and laughed with them. In them we see children full of life! Full of potential! Full of hope. We also see children on the brink; children whose lives are defined by adversity. We struggle with the concept of vulnerability because it's not African. We struggle because behind orphans and vulnerable children (OVC) is the sober reality of helplessness among children. This reality challenges us to take steps to understand their plight from what is known about them and from the children's own perspective. This book is an attempt at bringing this together in one place. It is also an invitation to dialogue, to reflect on the concept of vulnerability as an acceptable way of categorizing children. The book is a challenge and a call to action for all with power to positively influence the welfare of children, especially the welfare of the child living on the street, mourning the loss of a parent, heading a household—a sick, cold, and hungry child. We acknowledge Bishop Lombe, and men, women, and even children who are dedicated to accompanying children classified as vulnerable. We salute all who are committed to promoting human dignity, often under trying circumstances.

We are grateful for the opportunity to struggle with this issue. We express our sincere appreciation to friends and family who provided valuable support and feedback from the inception of this book to its completion. We are thankful to Yande for valuable conversations and support with organization of initial drafts. We appreciate the support provided by Grace Lombe, Protus Lumiti, and Nicholas Syano during the data collection and writing phases. We extend our sincere gratitude to everyone who took an interest in this work. We are deeply thankful to all contributors; this book would not have been written without your commitment to the welfare of children. We are especially indebted to children made vulnerable by HIV/AIDS in Botswana, Kenya, and Zambia, whose experiences this book draws upon. We thank them for their grace and courage in providing voice to their experiences; allowing us to see what life is like for them from their point of view. We truly appreciate the time and effort of all who made this work possible.

List of Abbreviations

ACRWC	African Charter on the Rights of the Child
AIDS	Acquired Immune Deficiency Syndrome
ARV	Antiretroviral
BAIS	Botswana AIDS Impact Survey
BOCONGO	Botswana Council of Non-Governmental Organizations
BWP	Botswana Pula
CBO	Community-Based Organization
CCN	Community Care Nigeria
COGRI	Children of God Relief Institute
CRC	Convention on the Rights of the Child
CSO	Central Statistics Office
DSS	Department of Social Services
FBOs	Faith-Based Organizations
HIV	Human Immunodeficiency Virus
IATT	Inter-Agency Task Team for Children affected by HIV/AIDS
MDGs	Millennium Development Goals
MLG	Ministry of Local Government
MOH	Ministry of Health
MTP	Medium Term Plan
NAP	National Action Plan
NGOs	Non-Governmental Organizations
OVC	Orphans and Vulnerable Children
PSS	Psychosocial Support Services
SADC	The Southern Africa Development Community
SLAs	Savings and Loans Associations
STPA	Short Term Plan of Action on the Care of Orphans
UNAIDS	United Nations Program on HIV/AIDS
UNICEF	United Nations Children's Emergency Fund
USAID	United States Agency for International Development

Introduction: Book Overview

Margaret Lombe and Harriet Mabikke

The issue of HIV/AIDS has received considerable attention worldwide. The past two decades have seen progress made on the scientific front. However, the dramatic consequence of the epidemic—especially in countries where access to prevention, treatment and care is severely limited—continues to grow. Sub-Saharan Africa is one of the regions that have been disproportionately impacted by the HIV/AIDS pandemic; losing a considerable proportion of adults in their most productive years. An aftermath of the high adult mortality rates has been an increase in the proportion of children who are orphaned. Indeed, approximately 9 out of 10 children classified as OVC worldwide live in this region alone. In light of the staggering toll of HIV/AIDS on the region, efforts have been made to curb the spread of the virus—mainly through treatment and prevention. These issues are important and compelling but fail to capture the whole picture; the unprecedented increase in the number of children classified as vulnerable. In response to this, during the past few years, individuals, communities and organizations—from a grandmother in a remote village to the policy-maker in the city—have risen to the challenge. Their effort in alleviating suffering among children classified as vulnerable is laudable. Despite this, children continue to experience high levels of vulnerability, provoking further dialogue.

Our modest contribution to this agenda is to highlight the plight of children in different living arrangements, review policies and interventions undertaken to enhance their welfare, identify gaps, if any, with respect to children's participation/visibility as well as awareness of human rights. These issues deserve attention because in the absence of well thought-out interventions that are guided by the voices of the primary stakeholder—affected children—children classified as vulnerable will continue to experience suffering and exploitation; negatively impacting their life chances and the wellbeing of communities. Moreover, we rest on the premise that society has a moral obligation to protect its vulnerable members, especially when they are children.

This book provides us with a platform from which to grapple with a number of issues including classification of young people who are subjects of rights as OVC, review of policies and interventions put in place to enhance their welfare, along with their perception of human rights.

On a practical note, the concept of OVC may be, and to some extent has been, an effective tool of highlighting the dilemma of children so classified; ensuring that they receive the much needed support. Yet again, what does vulnerability among children imply? In this group we have children affected/infected by HIV/AIDS, orphans, street children, children living in child-headed households, abandoned children, children with disabilities, displaced children, and children affected by armed conflict to mention a few. As such, the concept of OVC places various groups of children in one box, making a focused response difficult. Moreover, the concept of vulnerability itself may be problematic—*abalanda, mashikini* and *bana ba matshelo a bone a leng mo diphatseng* (in Bemba, Kiswahili and Setswana)—as it may confound the child's agency.[1] Throughout history, Africa, like any human society, has had to take care of vulnerable groups, including children, the poor, the sick and the elderly. In fact, strong familial and communal bonds are at the core of "Africaniness." We believe Africa has/had a term to define children that were orphaned and made vulnerable. What was that term? If indeed, the soul of society is revealed by the way it treats its children, what is the nature of Africa's soul?

The concept of OVC may be a depiction of the relationship that exist between the "helper" and "helpee" which defines the NGO culture. The "helpee" position, many Africans have assumed, may have contributed to the fragmentation of ubuntuism and loss of dignity. It may even have redefined how Africans relate to each other—especially to people considered vulnerable. In this relation, Africa may have lost its capacity to respond to the needy. When faced with challenges, its people extend open hands and look up to the "helper." Its people are swift to accept anything, even labels on Africa's children, in exchange for food and other hand-outs.

Labeling children as vulnerable, for these authors, is troubling. It may have negative/disempowering implications. Indeed, children so classified may internalize vulnerability, constraining their capacities, capabilities and structure of opportunity. Moreover, if we claim that children are our future, what does the future look like for sub-Saharan Africa? A future and legacy that rests on the shoulders of children classified as vulnerable! Our call is to re-imagine a world in which children classified as vulnerable can attain dignity and realize their full potential. This may require a different label, a label that springs from the primary stakeholders—the children themselves and their communities.

Another subject of concern is the acceptability and normalization of atypical or non-traditional living arrangements for children classified as vulnerable—e.g., in child-headed households, on streets and in orphanages. Before the AIDS epidemic consumed Africa, African communities nurtured and protected their children. Adult supervision was the norm; children were not left to fend for themselves, even for short periods. Yet, today, it has become acceptable for children to raise themselves. It's not uncommon for communities to proudly point out households headed by children to visitors. When did it become acceptable for children to head households?

---

1 Translations obtained from native speakers of the Bemba, Kiswahili and Setswana. It should be noted, however, that the people we spoke to found it difficult to identify the equivalent of the word "vulnerable," especially in Setswana.

In the same way, street children have become an acceptable feature of the African landscape. We know that many of the children in the streets have experienced the death of at least one parent. We recall an Africa where adults were duty-bound to protect and safeguard the welfare of children. Indeed, a child wandering the streets would be questioned and led to safety by a caring adult. Living on streets puts children classified as vulnerable at risk of various forms of exploitation, perpetuating the cycle of vulnerability. The fact that children are living on streets, sleeping under bridges and eating out of garbage bins is problematic and challenges the African spirit. We struggle with the idea of leaving children to fend for themselves on streets, hounded by adults and authority figures that are meant to protect them.

Furthermore, we question the acceptance of orphanages as a model of taking care of children classified as vulnerable. It is common knowledge that formal and informal organizations are involved in the running of orphanages in Africa without proper monitoring mechanisms; putting children at risk of abuse. In addition, well-meaning individuals tasked with the day-to-day operation of these facilities often lack the cultural sensitivity and knowledge needed to raise an African child. Moreover, there is some evidence to suggest that institutional care has detrimental effects on children and communities. In fact, in many parts of the world, institutional care has been abandoned in favor of family preservation. We believe that although many of the children in orphanages may have lost both parents, they still have the extended family. Given a choice and support, the extended familial system would elect to raise children classified as vulnerable at a fraction of the cost of operating orphanages and similar facilities.

Coupled with the other difficulties children classified as vulnerable are faced with, the African child in general, and OVC in particular, continue to be voiceless and invisible. Indeed, it is common knowledge that a child, in many African communities, is invisible—a non-participant—in the decision-making process at both the family and policy level. This is especially true for young people classified as vulnerable. Without a doubt, children in Africa are loved and nurtured. However, tradition has little regard for children's views and opinions. Indeed, many African cultures view children as objects of adults, perpetrating their invisibility and voicelessness, even in matters that affect them. Adages such as "a child is to be seen and not heard from," "children only speak when spoken to," and "children should not look adults in the eye," and other social norms that limit children's engagement in matters pertaining to their wellbeing, are not uncommon. At the death of a parent(s), for instance, orphaned children are rarely asked where or who they'd like to live with. In most cases they are separated from siblings so they do not even have each other for support.

Against this backdrop, the concept of human rights as they relate to the rights of the child may be problematic for an African child—children are nested in social structures that do not nurture/promote agency in children. Children often have limited knowledge of human rights and the protections these guarantee. Those that are aware of their rights often find it difficult to express their views freely out of fear of reprisal from communities and elders. Today, many African countries have put in place minimal mechanisms for children's participation in decision-making and governance, especially at the grassroots level. Moreover, governments/ countries commemorate June 16 as the day of the African child. Our challenge is to celebrate the African child each day by standing up for, and with, children classified as vulnerable. After all, this is the measure of society's greatness. It is also the right thing to do.

The predicament of children classified as vulnerable has revealed shortcomings in the moral fiber of African communities; one being the weakening of "ubuntuism"—the interconnectedness between humans or belief in the universal bond of sharing that connects all humanity. Society has witnessed, during the past few years, the slow demise of the communal spirit that characterizes Africa, this has been exemplified in social interaction with children classified as vulnerable. We have heard of adults engaged in the abuse of children, incidences of property grabbing—oftentimes undertaken by close relatives—are rampant, and, in addition, children are engaged in labor, at times under unsafe conditions for low pay. These challenges have necessitated continued dialogue. Where are the caring adults in this? How did the concept of OVC become normalized and acceptable? What about intergenerational transfer of social skills that defines human society, what is the source of these skills for children left to raise themselves? We believe the cycle of vulnerability can be broken. This is possible. Indeed, for years, African communities have demonstrated extraordinary capacity to rise above challenges (e.g., attainment of civil liberty, overcoming diseases, droughts, famines, and other environmental challenges), and have made gains in the use of technology. This book provides space to wrestle with issues experienced by children classified as vulnerable.

Scope of the Book

The book is divided into five main sections, covering nine distinctive chapters. Part I presents an overview of the HIV/AIDS pandemic in sub-Saharan Africa and its effect on children. The role of economic vulnerability in impacting life chances for children is addressed. Also presented is a synopsis of policies and programs put in place in response to the plight of vulnerable children in sub-Saharan Africa. Part II reviews the living arrangements of children in sub-Saharan Africa. This section is made up of three chapters addressing the situation of children in the three countries of focus: Botswana, Kenya and Zambia. Highlighted is the plight of children in supported facilities, foster care and child-headed households. The chapter on Botswana focuses on children in foster care. The chapter on Kenya addresses the situation of children in supported facilities. The chapter on Zambia deals with the situation of children in a variety of settings including child-headed households. Part III, consisting of three chapters, assesses governmental and community responses to the plight of children made vulnerable by the HIV/AIDS epidemic in sub-Saharan Africa. Implications for observed responses are discussed.

To fully capture the perception of the children and their vulnerable situation from the children's own perspective, Part IV supplements the literature reviewed with evidence from research conducted by the editors in Kenya and Zambia which targeted children in supported facilities as well as child-headed households (N = 187). Chapter 8 highlights seven key areas with regards to perceptions of children classified as vulnerable: (1) awareness of HIV/AIDS; (2) experiences within the home/institution or household; (3) relationship with family members; (4) relationship with community; (5) future orientation—goals and aspirations; (6) awareness of human rights as they relate to children; and (7) voice on treatment of children classified as vulnerable.

Part V, containing two chapters, situates the discussion within the context of human rights. Specifically, the meaning of vulnerability among children within the framework of the Convention on the Rights of the Child is examined. A synthesis of main arguments raised is presented in the final chapter.

PART I
Overview of the Issue

Chapter 1

AIDS-Related Vulnerability among Children in Sub-Saharan Africa: An Overview

Lyndsey McMahan, Chiedza Mufunde, and Margaret Lombe

Introduction and Background

The issue of HIV/AIDS has received considerable attention worldwide. The past two decades have seen progress made on the scientific front including tools and services aimed at prevention as well as treatment. Since 2011, the number of people worldwide newly infected with HIV and AIDS has decreased by 33 percent (UNAIDS, 2013). In addition, thanks to the development of life-saving antiretroviral therapies, the number of AIDS-related deaths have decreased from 2.3 million in 2005 to 1.6 million in 2012 (UNAIDS, 2013). However, the drastic consequence of the epidemic, especially in countries where access to prevention, treatment and care is severely limited, continues to grow. More than 20 years have passed since the first deaths from AIDS occurred. Most of these deaths occur in sub-Saharan Africa, one of the regions hardest hit by the epidemic. The disproportional loss of individuals in their most productive years raises concerns over the welfare of surviving members of affected families and social, political, and economic institutions. One consequence of the rapid increase in adult mortality is an increase in the proportion of children who are orphaned (Stover et al., 2008). According to AVERT (2005), at the end of 2001, an estimated 14 million children worldwide had lost a parent or both to AIDS or related causes. As of 2012, that number had reached 17.8 million (UNICEF, 2014). Sub-Saharan Africa accounts for nearly 90 percent of these orphans (UNICEF, 2014).

In recent years the phenomenon of orphans and vulnerable children (OVC) has received some attention in academic circles. However, there has not been stringent academic examination of the issue partly because the impact of the epidemic on children has proven to be particularly hard to quantify, confront, and even harder to put on the agendas of researchers. Due mainly to the staggering toll of HIV/AIDS, research effort has focused on treatment and prevention. Children have received attention mainly in relation to "mother to child transmission" and pediatric AIDS. These issues are important and compelling but fail to capture the whole story. The other part of this story is the orphan crisis that has engulfed the region in the past few years.

Before delving into the scope of the problem it is important to acknowledge the definition of OVC. According to Skinner et al. (2004), the term "orphaned and vulnerable children" was coined as a way of addressing the full scale problem of children orphaned by AIDS as well as those made vulnerable due to the epidemic and surrounding poverty. Although the term was created to be inclusive of all children, "it has no implicit definition or clear statement of inclusion and exclusion" (Skinner et al., 2004, p. 1). Further, vulnerability is difficult to define despite delineation of an implicit classification system for orphans including age of the child and nature of the caregiver (Skinner et al., 2006). In order for the definition of vulnerability to be inclusive, it must center around three core areas of child dependence: material problems, emotional problems, and social problems (Skinner et al., 2004). Table 1.1 presents a summary of the categories of children categorized as vulnerable in selected sub-Saharan countries.

Table 1.1 Definitions and differences of vulnerability regarding children in four African countries

Vulnerability	Zambia	South Africa	Botswana	Kenya
Truancy	x			
Female, older adult, or disabled headed households	x	x		
Terminally ill parent	x	x		x
Poor living conditions	x			
Child labor			x	
Sexual exploitation			x	
Neglect or abuse		x	x	
Unemployed caretakers		x		
Disabilities		x	x	x
Inconsistent access to resources	x		x	x
Indigenous minority			x	

Source: Created using data from Skinner et al., 2004, 2006 (p. 22).

According to UNICEF (2005), a child is considered vulnerable by HIV and AIDS if he or she is below the age of 18 and has lost one or both parents; has a chronically ill parent; lives in a household where at least one adult has died in the last 12 months and was sick for three months prior to death; or lives outside of family care. World Vision listed OVC identifiers as children who live in households that receive orphans or households with at least one person that is ill, dying, or deceased (Skinner et al., 2004). Based on these definitions and understandings of vulnerabilities, the term OVC is used to identify children below that age of 18 that have a differential access to resources which increases their insecurity and risk of danger due to causes related to HIV and AIDS (Schatz, 2009).

Sub-Saharan Africa is home to 56 million orphans, aged 0–17 years. About 15.1 million of these have been orphaned or made vulnerable by HIV and AIDS (UNICEF, 2014). Botswana, South Africa and Zambia have an estimated 15 percent or more children orphaned from AIDS (UNICEF, 2014). For many children, the impact of HIV and AIDS "engenders specific vulnerabilities such as the loss of parental care, food security, withdrawal from school, increased poverty, decreased access to healthcare, stigma, and increased risk of abuse and HIV infection" (Akwara et al., 2010). Indeed, Doku (2009) describes the state of AIDS orphans in Africa as the "orphan crisis," a crisis that puts millions of African children at heightened risk for physical, environmental, and psychosocial health problems.

The Plight of Vulnerable Children in Sub-Saharan Africa

According to Radcliff et al. (2012), children born in Africa are at greater risks of problems than their counterparts born in other parts of the world. One of the greatest struggles that children who are orphaned or made vulnerable by HIV face is poverty. Poverty and HIV often coexist, and where they do, children become at risk for greater deprivation (UNICEF, 2006). According to Murphy (2008), the AIDS epidemic threatens traditional resource management systems because adult labor and knowledge is often lost. When a member of the household becomes sick from HIV or AIDS there is often a decrease in income because of the caregiver's inability to work and an increase in medical related expenses (UNICEF, 2006). Because children are actors within households and not mere recipients of adult care (Ansell and Blerk, 2004), these two factors often compromise a child's welfare. For example, children in households where caretakers become sick are at greater risk of food insecurity because the adults are less capable of participating in subsistence activities. Children need an adequate supply of food in order to prevent developmental delays in growth and diseases associated with poor nutrition (Radcliff et al., 2012). In addition to physical aspects, poor nutrition can also cause psychosocial issues, poor emotional wellbeing, and poor educational outcomes (Radcliff et al., 2012).

Although many of the vulnerabilities that children face are poverty related, migration is a factor that many children and caregivers must face as a result of HIV and AIDS. Migration, which is often seen as a source of strength in sub-Saharan Africa, often increases the dependency ratio[1] in households that already do not have adequate resources to care for their own members (UNICEF, 2006). Households with orphans generally have the highest dependency ratios, with female-headed households having the highest of all (UNICEF, 2006). In sub-Saharan Africa 22.4 percent of children live in households where they are not the offspring of the

1 The dependency ratio is the number of children aged 0–17 plus the number of adults over the age of 60 divided by the number of adults aged 18–59 (UNICEF, 2006).

household heads and at least 31 percent of these children have moved more than once (Ansell and Blerk, 2004).

Migration experiences for children classified as vulnerable are often complex, and although generally prompted by AIDS, are far from being a straightforward process (Ansell and Young, 2004). Most children find that the act of migration can be not only traumatic in the short term but these experienced traumas can carry over to the long term due to the difficulties of adjusting to new communities and social groups (Ansell and Young, 2004). Webb argues that there is an increasingly assumed relationship between orphanhood and AIDS which exacerbates problems that OVCs face regarding integration into communities (as cited in Ansell and Young, 2004). Children who are forced to migrate often are not aware of the reasons why their family members were sick and subsequently are not informed about the reasons for migration which increases their anxiety around the move (Ansell and Young, 2004). Child-rearing in sub-Saharan Africa is traditionally vested in families and to some extent extended families, making migration experiences in some countries, such as Zambia, confusing because they are largely patrilineal societies (Ansell and Blerk, 2004; NAC, 2012). According to Ansell and Blerk (2004), in patrilineal societies it might be expected that "where the mother was married, paternal relatives would care for orphaned children. The choice of guardian was, however, often made on pragmatic grounds: if paternal grandparents were too old or too poor, maternal grandparents or other relatives were preferred" (p. 681). Although there is a predominant patrilineal make-up in a number of sub-Saharan countries, there are others, such as Malawi, that tend to be less culturally homogeneous and divide between patrilineal and matrilineal traditions (Ansell and Blerk, 2004).

Although migration is sometimes seen as a coping skill for parents that are living with HIV, evidence shows that children who have migrated to new households often experience discrimination regarding allocation of resources (UNICEF, 2006). Children who are not direct biological descendants of the heads of households often receive different or less food than other children, are beaten and overworked, and receive inadequate clothing (UNICEF, 2006). Ansell and Young (2004) state that "when households adopt children through a sense of obligation, as is usually the case with AIDS orphans, they are often treated differently from the family's 'biological' children, particularly if resources are scarce" (p. 5). For example, children who migrate and consequently live in foster situations are often expected to work in order to contribute to the wage earnings of their new households (Ansell and Young, 2004). A child so affected may experience poor education outcomes since access to school may be negatively affected as money typically used to meet school expenses is spent on other things. The time that would primarily be spent in schools or on leisure is now required to help with household chores and subsistence activities (Richter, 2004). Children in this situation often experience extreme stress, heightening the potential for abnormal or delayed psychosocial development (Richter, 2004). Factors such as these have a great impact on the orphan school attendance ratio,[2] which is much higher in countries such as Kenya, Zambia, and Botswana that have higher rates of orphans.

Although psychosocial development happens throughout the lifespan, in the early years there is an interaction between genetics, attachment, and daily experiences which helps to shape personalities and vulnerabilities (Elegbeleye, 2013). "The consequences of poor mental health in childhood extend into adulthood, increasing the likelihood of low education achievement, reduced productivity, criminality and violence, adult mental disorder, unhealthy lifestyles and the risk of ill health" (Elegbeleye, 2013, p. 172). This means that in order for children to experience normal psychosocial development, factors within their micro-systems must be working together in order to enhance and promote the early experiences. Risk factors such as food insecurity, migration, and fostering leave OVC at great risk for poor mental health because they do not achieve their full potential for behavioral, social, and cognitive development (Elegbeleye, 2013). Although these risk factors increase the likelihood that OVC will develop a mental illness, another struggle that orphaned and vulnerable children must face is stigma. Stigma can be defined as a "deeply discrediting attribute that reduces a person to someone who is in some way tainted and can therefore be denigrated" (Skinner and Mfecane, 2004). It is generally understood that the psychological and physical wellbeing of children who are stigmatized will be threatened by further excluding them from resources and support (Skinner and Mfecane, 2004). Stigma also increases the likelihood that orphaned and vulnerable children will experience anxiety and depression. According to Ansell and Blerk (2004), in sub-Saharan Africa, adults or other caregivers do not often believe that children suffer from emotional problems and do not understand the grief that OVC experience.

The psychological impact of HIV and AIDS as well as factors associated with them is often overlooked in regards to, not only children, but caregivers as well (Salaam, 2004). According to Salaam (2004), it is not uncommon for senior citizens that have no social security or retirement benefits to care for a dozen children at once—a phenomenon referred to as grandparent-headed households. Not only does this leave the caregivers exhausted and in a state of toxic stress but it also increases the likelihood that the children will be uneducated and malnourished (Salaam, 2004). In addition to being uneducated and malnourished, AIDS-orphaned adolescents in such households have been shown to be at risk for mental health problems, depression, peer problems, post-traumatic stress, and behavior problems (Cluver et al., 2008). These risk factors leave older caregivers in even more stress, making it difficult to provide adequate care for those made vulnerable by HIV or AIDS.

---

2 "The orphan school attendance ratio is the ratio of the percentage of children 10–14 years old who have lost both parents and are currently attending school to the percentage of non-orphaned children of the same age, both of whose parents are alive and who are living with at least one parent and attending school" (UNICEF, 2010, p. 22).

Responses to the Plight of Vulnerable Children in Sub-Saharan Africa

The lasting and negative impact of vulnerability caused by HIV/AIDS has prompted a need for interventions to respond to this crisis. Various programs, interventions, and policies have been established to meet the needs of children and families affected by the AIDS pandemic. Understanding the social environment that shapes a child's life is important in shaping these responses. The social structures, such as family and kinship, religion, education system, government and healthcare system, in which a child exists, help to define who that child becomes (Hutchison, 2008). Indeed, in order for a child to develop properly each sector of the child's life must work together. When a child exists in an environment that is supportive and loving then that child is more likely to receive cognitive and social stimulation, enhancing his or her chances to succeed in school and ultimately in life (Chilton, 2007). This group effort becomes part of the collective agency in which people act together to meet needs and accomplish goals (Hutchison, 2011).

According to UNICEF (2006), "the age of orphans and their age when they were orphaned, have significant implications for planning a response that meets children's needs at varying developmental stages" (p. 6). Since the majority of orphans and vulnerable children depend on their families and communities, there is a need for integrated approaches that simultaneously address the needs of children, caregivers, and communities. Recognizing these interventions that offer financial assistance, emergency support for families caring for vulnerable children, and child-headed households is critical (Salaam, 2004).

Scholarly and programmatic responses to rights and needs of orphans across Africa have been active at the community, national, and international level. The responses are varied within and across the identified levels. Communities have been actively taking collective responsibility in taking care of children who lose their parents to AIDS. The support at the community level has been facilitated through families and religious organizations. At the global level, several working groups and inter-agency alliances have convened to find the best solutions to improve lives of orphans and vulnerable children globally. An overview of policies and programs that have been put in place to advance the welfare of OVC in sub-Saharan Africa are presented below.

International Response

Concern over the growing number of orphans led to a consensus on the "Framework for the Protection, Care and Support of Orphans and Vulnerable Children Living in a World with HIV and AIDS." This tool, known as "The Framework" (see Figure 1.1), was developed in 2004 by the Global Partners Forum on Children Affected by HIV and AIDS with leadership from the UNAIDS Committee (UNICEF, 2011; Save the Children, 2010). Guidelines emerging from The Framework provide policies as well as a programmatic basis to achieve goals set for orphans and other children

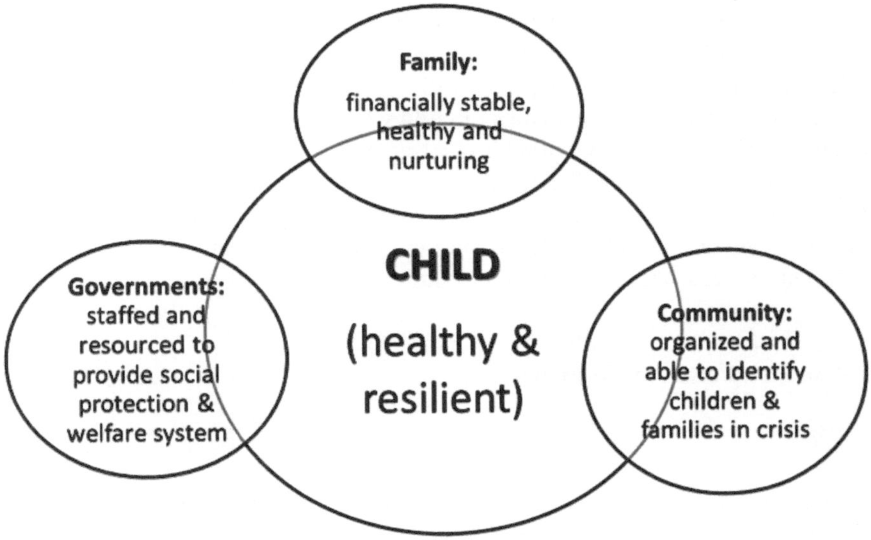

Figure 1.1 "The Framework"
Source: Adapted from G. Bachman, UNICEF, 2011.

made vulnerable by AIDS. The core strategies outlined in "The Framework" aim to: (1) strengthen the capacity of families; (2) mobilize community-based responses to vulnerable households; (3) increase orphans' access to essential services; (4) ensure government protection through improved policy and legislation; and (5) raise awareness at all levels through advocacy and social mobilization (UNICEF, 2004). It is against this backdrop that countries hit hardest by the AIDS epidemic and subsequent escalation in the number of OVC, established the National Action Plans on Orphaned and Vulnerable Children. It should also be noted that The Framework is heavily influenced by the Convention on the Rights of the Child, 2001 United Nations Special Session on HIV and AIDS, and the 2002 United Nations General Assembly Special Session on Children (Save the Children, 2010). Therefore, The Framework has become an important reference point for policies and programming in response to the plight of orphans and vulnerable children in sub-Saharan Africa and beyond.

In addition to "The Framework," another global multi-agency network of over 50 organizations was created under UNICEF. The Inter-Agency Task Team for Children affected by HIV/AIDS (IATT) addresses the need to strengthen national systems for OVC by promoting harmonization of policy guidance and programming. The IATT also promotes the development and sharing of technical and programmatic information among stakeholders (UNICEF, n.d.). Furthermore, the United States President's Emergency Plan for AIDS Relief (PEPFAR), launched in 2003, has been instrumental in the overall fight against HIV/AIDS and support for children affected and made vulnerable by the epidemic. PEPFAR recognizes the central importance and care for OVC as necessary complement to biomedical efforts to end HIV/AIDS (Nyberg et al., 2012). The 2006 PEPFAR OVC Guidance identified six fundamental domains of child wellbeing: education, health, shelter and care, food and nutrition, psychosocial support and protection from abuse and neglect, plus improving families' ability to provide for a child's needs (Nyberg et al., 2012). After years of supporting programs across sub-Saharan Africa, PEPFAR has been utilizing a multi-sectoral and multi-disciplinary interaction to address child/family needs that are context-specific.

National and/or Local Responses

Policies

The National Action Plans (NAPs) for Orphans and Vulnerable Children have been widely adopted across sub-Saharan Africa within relevant ministries. Improved policy and legislation is an essential component in improving service provision for OVC; by the end of 2010, 17 countries in Eastern and Southern Africa were in the process of strengthening and developing comprehensive NAPs (Save the Children, 2010). Botswana, Kenya, and Zambia are some of the countries with a comprehensive plan to support OVC and fight AIDS. The level of impact through these policy plans varies across the continent. The 2011–15 National HIV and AIDS Strategic Framework by the Zambian government articulates the urgency for prevention and care for the most vulnerable children (National HIV and AIDS Strategic Framework, 2010). Support for households with children made vulnerable by AIDS has been the most challenging, with about 20 percent of households receiving support in Zambia (see Figure 1.2). Botswana is an example of a country that has implemented a 10-year NAP and has identified the need for a national policy regarding OVC that includes access to medical and material assistance as well as programs that address psychosocial support, behavior management, and child welfare (Department of Social Services, 2009).

As outlined in Figure 1.2, Botswana has the largest number of households receiving support from the government and other entities supporting OVC. A well-implemented strategic framework on OVC is critical in developing interventions and programs for families in need. Lastly, in Kenya, the level of support for households with OVC increased between 2006 and 2008—this increase can be attributed to the additional policies to support OVC within the larger national framework on HIV/AIDS in Kenya where 12 of all children are orphaned by AIDS (National AIDS Control Council, 2009). Lessons from the development and implementation of NAPs for OVC are illustrative, and point to the need to mainstream responses to OVC needs within broader policies and plans for children, HIV, social protection, poverty reduction and other social instruments (UNICEF, 2011).

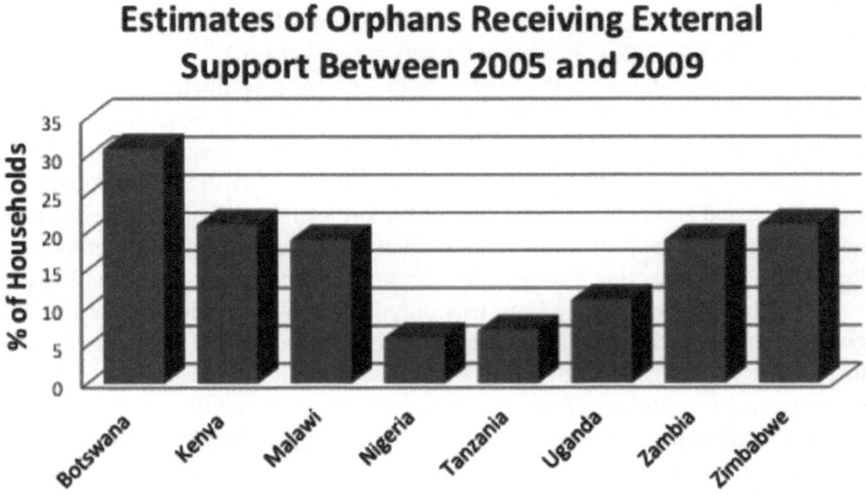

Figure 1.2 Percentage of orphans receiving external support
Source: Created using data from UNICEF ChildInfo.org, 2011.

Programs

A number of programs have been put in place in response to the needs of OVC. A brief overview of these is presented below.

Jali Watoto, Tanzania
There are several community-based interventions working with rural communities affected by HIV/AIDS. The SAWAKA *Jali Watoto* (Care for Children) program in Kagera, Tanzania is one example of an effective model for working with vulnerable children and their caregivers. The *Jali Watoto* model recognizes the dramatic changes that children affected by HIV go through. This program is aimed at mitigating the impact on the children's emotional and physical health (Nyangara et al., 2009). The intervention focuses on community support, sensitization, mobilization, and advocacy, and is aimed at strengthening the capacity and response to the needs of the most vulnerable children and their families (Nyangara et al., 2009). The program creates a safe and supportive environment for community members because the community takes ownership of the programs which allows them to reflect their local needs. In addition to the support network that is formed, SAWAKA *Jali Watoto* also provides educational, counselling and medical support to the children and caregivers.

Community Care Nigeria
Community Care Nigeria (CCN) was a three-year OVC program developed by Christian Aid that focused on the capacity building of families and communities

in order for them to provide more effective services to orphans and vulnerable children (USAID, 2007). The program was active between 2007 and 2010, and offered targeted support in the core domains of child wellbeing. The program worked with children of all ages and adults over 18 years who were affected or living with HIV. Through the Savings and Loans Associations (SLAs), Community Care strengthened households with methods of saving, obtaining small loans and access to financial support. Adolescents received health education and psychosocial support to overcome trauma, food and nutrition incorporating local diets, and protection through OVC committees addressing stigma and abuse.

Even though Community Care was only active over a three-year period, the goals of the project aimed at making a lasting impact in the eight rural states in Nigeria. As a result, 11,875 OVC were reached and they receive more than two services. In addition, 77 percent of households are benefiting from SLAs and 80 community-based facilitators were trained to support families. This model is promising as a catalyst for strengthening local capacity and within families as well as connecting families to services available to them (AIDSTAR-One, n.d.).

Mama Mkubwa Psychosocial Support Group, Tanzania

Implemented by the Salvation Army, Mama Mkubwa is an exemplary community-based initiative of volunteer committees that identify vulnerable children and families. This model is an example of a community responding to local needs. This community-based program focuses on community sensitization and mobilization with the aim to strengthen community capacity and response to needs of OVC and their families through psychosocial support (AIDSTAR-One, n.d.). Some of the core activities carried out by Mama Mkubwa committees include kids' clubs for children aged 2–12. These clubs meet on a regular basis and are open to all children within the community. In addition to the children's clubs, committees also receive training and ongoing support regarding community counselling as a way of sensitizing the community on the needs of OVC.

Key achievements of this intervention include the central involvement of community leaders which ensures sustainability of the program. Furthermore, the community-based action planning reduces dependence on the Salvation Army, fosters ownership and unites the community. Most importantly, this model relies on community members to choose beneficiaries for the program, hence capitalizing on local knowledge of vulnerability (AIDSTAR-One, n.d.). An evaluation of Mama Mkubwa identified the need for developing the necessary skills and capacity for the community members involved with this program. This will ensure that members of the committees involved do not get burned out, but can remain committed and able to carry out this critical role in supporting OVC (Littrell et al., 2007).

ARK Model, South Africa

Nurturing Orphans of AIDS for Humanity (NOAH) was established in 2000 as a response to the overwhelming number of orphaned children in South Africa. In

South Africa 19.6 percent, or roughly 3.6 million children, are orphaned of which half of these are orphaned by AIDS (NOAH Community, n.d.). NOAH has more than 10 partner organizations (local and international) offering support to OVC from infancy to 17 years. This 10-step program calls for motivated individuals and leaders from a community to set up their own network of care for their OVC. The network, known as an Ark, includes a community committee of stakeholders and volunteers who develop a community-owned resource center. Ark committees are independent, but receive ongoing support from NOAH. Services provided include birth registration, home visits, accessing grants, food gardens, and feeding schemes.

Through NOAH, more than 29,000 orphans have been receiving support through Ark-based initiatives in KwaZulu Natal and Gauteng provinces. In 2009, NOAH was active in 105 communities with 30,318 registered children and more than 20,000 of them were receiving at least three of the core services (NOAH Community, n.d.). Similar to the *Mama Mkubwa* and *Jali Watoto* models, the *Ark* model also utilizes the participatory approach, community involvement, working with local leaders, and focuses on self-reliance and psychosocial support—this approach strengthens community responsibility in solving local problems. Furthermore, the independent nature of the Ark committees enables communities to tailor their community centers to the local needs of orphans and vulnerable children.

Conclusion

As outlined throughout this chapter, children orphaned or made vulnerable by HIV and AIDS face considerable challenges. The external experiences throughout a child's life course carry a serious and powerful weight that affects both their development and overall welfare (Bragin, 2012). "Orphanhood by AIDS has been associated with depression, delinquency, conduct problems, stigmatization, and post-traumatic stress" (Kirkpatrick et al., 2012). In addition to these, OVC must face not only the loss of their parents but the challenges of abuse related to migration and fostering, poverty, and cultural silence[3] (Thamuku and Daniel, 2013). Children are continually changed by how they experience their realities and this changed knowledge must be explored and engaged in order to help children, caretakers, and communities move forward (Bragin, 2012).

The interventions in response to the rights and needs of children classified as vulnerable interact at the various levels, with support from national and international non-governmental and governmental institutions. Most notably, economic and social rights are the human rights most central to the development of a child; the social structures, such as family and kinship, religion, education

3 Cultural silence refers to the taboos regarding the discussion of death, sex, and other related issues with children (Thamuku and Daniel, 2013).

system, government, and healthcare system, in which a child exists, help to define who that child becomes (Chilton, 2007; Hutchison, 2008). Therefore, responses to these challenges require holistic and targeted interventions that build capacity for families and communities to meet these challenges. However, communities cannot face these challenges alone. National and global efforts are critical in mobilizing the fight against HIV and improving the lives of children left behind due to AIDS. The state of orphaned and vulnerable children varies across sub-Saharan Africa therefore responses ought to be tailored to the specific challenges in the different countries. Programs outlined in this chapter are evidence of the power of family and community-based interventions in mobilizing strengths within the community as well as sensitizing caregivers to the challenges of OVC. Furthermore, the national-level policies and programs are essential in supporting the functioning of the community-based interventions for OVC. At the global level, OVC issues continue to be on the global agenda with influential international agencies such as the United Nations, UNICEF, and UNAIDS.

The 2004 "Framework for the Protection, Care and Support of Orphans and Vulnerable Children Living in a World with HIV and AIDS" has been the guiding light for national-based policies for OVC in countries affected by the AIDS crisis. "The Framework" is critical because it is inspired by the principles from the Convention on the Rights of the Child. The rights-based approach to the challenges affecting children orphaned by AIDS is critical in designing programs and interventions for these children: they are children, first; but have been made vulnerable by AIDS, and governments have the duty to fulfill the rights of the millions of children. Society has the responsibility to ensure children defined as vulnerable realize their optimal development and potential.

Bibliography

Africa (n.d.). Index Mundi. http://www.indexmundi.com/africa.html.

AIDSTAR-One (n.d.). http://www.aidstar-one.com/.

Akwara, P.A., Noubary, B., Ah Ken, P.L., et al. (2010). Who is the vulnerable child? Using survey data to identify children at risk in the era of HIV and AIDS. *AIDS Care*, 22(9), 1066–85.

Ansell, N. and Blerk, L.V. (2004). Children's migration as a household/family strategy: Coping with AIDS in Lesotho and Malawi. *Journal of Southern African Studies*, 30(3), 673–90.

Ansell, N. and Young, L. (2004). Enabling households to support successful migration of AIDS orphans in southern Africa. *AIDS Care*, 16(1), 3–10.

AVERT (2005). *Providing Drug Treatment for Millions*. West Sussex: Avert.

Bragin, M. (2012). Editorial. Special issue on children affected by armed conflict: Views from the global south. *International Journal of Applied Psychoanalytic Studies*, 9(3), 179–86.

Chilton, M., Chyatte, M., and Breaux, J. (2007). The negative effects of poverty and food insecurity on child development. *Indian Journal of Medical Research*, 126(4), 262–72.

Cluver, L.D., Gardner, F., and Operario, D. (2008). Effects of stigma on the mental health of adolescents orphaned by AIDS. *Journal of Adolescent Health*, 42, 410–17.

Community Care in Nigeria (CCN) (n.d.). AIDSTAR-One. http://www.aidstarone.com/promising_practices_database/g3ps/community_care_nigeria_ccn.

Department of Social Services (2010). *Botswana National Plan of Action for Orphans and Vulnerable Children, 2010–2016*. Gaborone, Botswana: Author.

Doku, P.N. (2009). Parental HIV/AIDS status and death, and children's psychological wellbeing. *International Journal of Mental Health Systems*, 3(26), http://doi.org/10.1186/1752-4458-3-26.

Doku, P.N. (2010). Parental AIDS status and death: Its impact on Ghanaian childrens' psychological well-being. *Nigerian Journal of Psychiatry*, 8(2), 24–31.

Elegbeleye, A. (2013). Predictors of the mental health of orphans and vulnerable children in Nigeria. *Ife Psychologia*, 21(2), 170–80.

Hutchison, E.D. (2008). Social institutions and social structure. In E.D. Hutchison (ed.), *Dimensions of Human Behavior: Person and Environment* (pp. 297–346). Thousand Oaks: Sage Publications.

Hutchison, E.D. (2011). A life course perspective. In E.D. Hutchison (ed.), *Dimensions of Human Behavior: The Changing Life Course* (pp. 1–38). Thousand Oaks: Sage Publications.

IATT CABA (2010). Stigma Action Network. http://www.iattcaba.org/web/guest/about-us.

Kirkpatrick, S., Rojjanasrirat, W., South, B., et al. (2012). Assessment of emotional status of orphans and vulnerable children in Zambia. *Journal of Nursing Scholarship*, 44(2), 194–201.

Littrell, M., Thurman T.R., Chatterji, M., and Brown, L. (2007). *Mama Mkubwa Psychosocial Program: A Case Study*. Chapel Hill, NC: MEASURE Evaluation.

Murphy, L. (2008). AIDS and kitchen gardens: Insights from a village in western Kenya. *Population and Environment*, 29(3/5), 133–61.

National AIDS Control Council (2009). *Kenya National AIDS Strategic Plan 2009/10–2012/13: Delivering on Universal Access to Services*. Nairobi, Kenya: Author.

National AIDS Coordinating Agency, The (2009). *The Second National Strategic Framework for HIV and AIDS: 2010–2016*. Gaborone: Ministry of State President.

National AIDS Council (NAC) (2012). *Zambia Country Report: Monitoring the Declaration of Commitment on HIV and AIDS and the Universal Access* (biennial report). Republic of Zambia: Author.

National HIV and AIDS Strategic Framework (2010). *National AIDS Strategic Framework 2011–2015: Towards Improving the Quality of Life of the Zambian People*. Lusaka, Zambia: Author.

NOAH Community (n.d.). http://www.noahcommunity.org/.

Nyangara, F. and Obiero, W. (2009). Effects of a community-focused approach supporting the most vulnerable children: Evaluation of SAWAKA *Jali Watoto* program in Kagera, Tanzania. MEASURE Evaluation. http://www.cpc.unc.edu/measure/publications/sr-09-55.

Nyberg, B.J., Yates, D.D., Lovich, R., et al. (2012). Saving lives for a lifetime: Supporting orphans and vulnerable children impacted by HIV/AIDS. *JAIDS Journal of Acquired Immune Deficiency Syndromes*, 60, S127–S135.

PEPFAR (2006). Orphans and Other Vulnerable Children Programming Guidance for United States Government In-Country Staff and Implementing Partners. http://www.pepfar.gov/documents/organization/83298.pdf.

Radcliff, E., Racine, E., Huber, L.B., and Whitaker, B. (2012). Association between family composition and the well-being of vulnerable children in Nairobi, Kenya. *Maternal Child Health Journal*, 16, 1232–40.

Richter, L. (2004). The impact of HIV/AIDS on the development of children [monograph]. *A Generation at Risk? HIV/AIDS, Vulnerable Children and Security in Southern Africa*, 109, 9–31.

Richter, L.M., Sherr, L., Adato, M., et al. (2009). Strengthening families to support children affected by HIV and AIDS. *AIDS Care*, 21(S1), 3–12.

Salaam, T. (2004). AIDS orphans and vulnerable children (OVC): Problems, responses, and issues for Congress. *Congressional Research Service*, RL32252, 1–24.

Save the Children (2010). *Establishing reviewing and implementing national plans of action for orphans and vulnerable children in Southern and East Africa: lessons learnt and challenges.* London, UK: Author.

Schatz, E.J. (2009). Reframing vulnerability: Mozambican refugees' access to state-funded pensions in rural South Africa. *Journal of Cross Cultural Gerontology*, 24, 241–58.

Skinner, D. and Mfecane, S. (2004). Stigma, discrimination and the implications for people living with HIV/AIDS in South Africa. *Journal of Social Aspects of HIV/AIDS*, 1(3), 157–64.

Skinner, D., Tsheko, N., Mtero-Munyati, S., et al. (2004). *Defining Orphaned and Vulnerable Children*. Cape Town: Human Sciences Research Council.

Skinner, D., Tsheko, N., Mtero-Munyati, S., et al. (2006). Towards a definition of orphaned and vulnerable children. *AIDS Behavior*, 10, 619–26.

Stover, J., Fidzani, B., Molomo, B.C., et al. (2008). Estimated HIV trends and program effects in Botswana. *PLoS ONE*, 3(11): e3729.

Thamuku, M. and Daniel, M. (2013). Exploring responses to transformative group therapy for orphaned children in the context of mass orphaning in Botswana. *Death Studies*, 37(5), 413–47.

UNAIDS (2009). The interagency task team on children and HIV and AIDS, 1–4. http://www.unicef.org/aids/files/ToR_IATT_2009.doc.

UNAIDS (2013). *Global Report: UNAIDS Report on the Global AIDS Epidemic*. Geneva: Author.

UNICEF (n.d.). UNICEF Partners and Networks. http://www.unicef.org/aids/index_iatt.html.

UNICEF (2004). The framework for the protection, care and support of orphans and vulnerable children living in a world with HIV and AIDS. Technical and Policy Documents. http://www.unicef.org/aids/files/Framework_English.pdf.
UNICEF (2005). *Guide to Monitoring and Evaluation of the National Response for Children Orphaned and made Vulnerable by HIV/AIDS*. New York: UNICEF.
UNICEF (2006). *Africa's Orphaned and Vulnerable Generations: Children Affected by AIDS*. New York: UNICEF.
UNICEF (2007). *Enhanced Protection for Children Affected by AIDS—A Companion Paper to The Framework for the Protection, Care and Support of Orphans and Vulnerable Children Living in a World with HIV and AIDS*. New York: UNICEF.
UNICEF (2010). *Children and AIDS: 5th Stocktaking Report*. New York: UNICEF, 1–52.
UNICEF (2011). Taking evidence to impact: Making a difference for vulnerable children living in a world with HIV and AIDS, 1–78. http://www.unicef.org/eapro/TAKING_EVIDENCE_TO_IMPACT_FINAL.pdf.
UNICEF (2014). The state of the world's children in numbers: Every child counts, 1–116. http://www.unicef.org/sowc2014/numbers/documents/english/SOWC 2014_In%20Numbrs_28%20Jan.pdf.
USAID (2007). New insights on preventing child marriage: A global analysis of factors and programs.

PART II
The Living Arrangements of Orphaned and Vulnerable Children in Sub-Saharan Africa

Part II reviews the living arrangements of children in sub-Saharan Africa. Highlighted are the living arrangements of children in formally supported facilities, foster care, as well as child-headed households. It is organized into three chapters; each chapter opens with a country background. The characteristics and situation of OVC in each country are also reviewed. Unless otherwise stated, the definition of OVC articulated by UNICEF is utilized. Acknowledging the complexity of the issue of OVC and challenges faced by children in this group, each chapter focuses on context-specific features.

Chapter 2 examines the tradition of fostering as well as the situation of fostered children in Botswana. It also highlights experiences of fostered children and those of their caregivers. Legal frameworks guiding fostering are explored. The chapter concludes with a discussion of challenges inherent in the foster care system and how these could be rectified.

Chapter 3 reviews the situation of children in residential care in Kenya. The children's characteristics are highlighted along with the complexity of the issue of OVC care and challenges faced by children in this group. The Children of God Relief Institute (COGRI) which includes Nyumbani Children's Home in Karen, Nairobi and Nyumbani Village in Kitui, Machakos County is utilized to frame this discussion.

Finally, Chapter 4 highlights different living arrangements of children in Zambia. An outline of children in single-parent households, households headed by a grandparent, foster care, orphanages, and other supported facilities is presented. Challenges experienced by children in child-headed households are specifically underscored. Policies and legal frameworks that safeguard the welfare of orphaned and vulnerable children are also explored. Overall, the section shows that communities have responded to the needs of vulnerable children using different arrangements of care. Although governmental initiatives exist, the system of care, for the most part, has been informal, relying on traditional networks.

Chapter 2
Fostered Children in Botswana

Tapologo Maundeni, Naomi Seboni, and Ogar Rapinyana

Introduction and Background Information: Country Profile

Botswana is a landlocked country in Southern Africa. It shares its borders with almost all Southern African countries, namely, South Africa (South), Namibia (West), Zimbabwe (North East), Angola (North West), and Zambia (North East). Its surface area is large compared to its population. It has an area of 570,000 km^2, around the same size as France or the state of Texas in the United States. Botswana, formerly known as Bechuanaland Protectorate, was a former colony of the British government from 1886 until 1966 when it gained its independence from the British government. Unlike other former colonies, it was not developed by its colonizers. At independence it was classified among the 10 poorest countries in the world.

Botswana has a relatively homogeneous small population of approximately two million (Central Statistics Office, 2013). The majority of Batswana belong to the Tswana ethnic group. Other ethnic groups include the Basarwa, Bayei, Bakalanga, and Bakgalagadi, amongst others. These have their own indigenous cultures and languages. A significant proportion of the country's population resides in the fertile and arable eastern bend, while the rest of the country is sparsely populated. In 2001, it was estimated that about 80 percent of the population resided in the rural area (Central Statistics Office, 2001). However, by 2007, about 60 percent of the population lived in rural areas compared to 40 percent who live in urban areas (Central Statistics Office, 2009). Generally, the population of Botswana is predominately made up of youth; today, the picture remains unchanged. Young people, between the ages of 10 and 29 years, account for 60 percent of the population. It is therefore critical to recognize their comprehensive needs/problems, in particular, their sexual and reproductive health and rights, and to address them adequately.

Botswana is a democratic country with a multiparty political system. Elections have been held every five years since 1966. The country enjoys political and economic stability and is often referred to as a model of democracy in Africa. Rapid development has benefitted most of Botswana's population. However, the country suffers from issues such as poverty and an increase in existing and emerging chronic diseases such as HIV and AIDS, tuberculosis, and cancer. Approximately 30 percent of the population live under the poverty datum line (Central Statistics Office, 2005). Poverty has disproportionately affected female-headed households, which accounted for 47 percent of the households in the country—52 percent of these were in the rural areas (Government of Botswana, 2008a; UNDP, 2012). The HIV national prevalence rate was estimated at 17.6 percent in 2008 (Central Statistics Office, 2009) compared to 17.1 percent in 2004. Current estimates stand at 18.5 percent (Republic of Botswana, 2013).

The country is relatively wealthy and boasts of minerals such as diamonds, coal, copper, and nickel. In fact, Botswana's wealth has increased relatively over the years and it is now classified as a middle-income country. Infrastructure, including communication, transportation, and road networks, has been established within the country and the SADC region (Government of Botswana, 2008a). This has facilitated movement of people from the highly populated eastern parts to remote areas such as the Kalahari Desert. It is important to note that the people of Botswana are highly mobile; families usually have three to four different homes in: (1) the city (*teropo*); (2) the village (*motse/legae*); (3) the ploughing place (*masimo*); and (4) the place where cattle are reared (*moraka*).

The living arrangements, characterized by seasonal movement, although culturally defined, have created major risks for children as they are often left unsupervised by an adult. Also, these patterns of living tend to pose a challenge to the healthcare system. Indeed, seasonal movement has facilitated the spread of HIV/AIDS and other communicable diseases, and has made caregiving and follow-up for those with chronic illnesses difficult.

Definition of Concepts

It is important to define the main concepts captured in the title of this chapter, namely child, orphan, and vulnerability. There are several definitions of the child according to different policies in Botswana. The definitions of a child differ in terms of the purpose for which such a definition is made, and at times these definitions are contradictory. The Children's Act of 2009 and the African Charter on the Rights and Welfare of the Child of 1999 define a child as anyone aged 18 years and below. The Adoption Act of 1952 on the other hand defines a child as a person aged 19 years and below. These stipulations suggest that a person who has sexual intercourse with a child aged 16 years and under will be charged with defilement. This interpretation may be problematic. By implication, it means that a child aged between 17 and 21 years is mature enough to consent to sexual intercourse. In contrast, a young person is defined as anyone aged 12 to 29 years (National Youth Policy, 1996). Further, Botswana delineates the age of maturity as 21 years (Botswana Constitution). These conflicting definitions may impact negatively on the decisions regarding child rights and protection in this country.

Unlike that of a child, the definitions of an orphan by different authorities appear to be relatively consistent. UNICEF/UNAIDS (1999) defines an orphan as a child under 15 years of age who has lost their mother (maternal orphan) or both parents (double orphan) to AIDS. Orphans are also defined by the Ministry of Local Government (1999) as any child aged 18 years and below, who has lost one or both biological parents. The Ministry of Local Government (2008) expanded on the above definition to include those children aged 18 years and below who have lost adoptive parents. Another unique label is that of social orphans: These are viewed as those children who have been neglected and abandoned by parents who cannot be traced (Ministry of Local Government, 1999).

With regards to vulnerability, the Ministry of Local Government (2008) defines "a vulnerable child as a person under the age of 18 years who is in any situation or circumstance which is or likely to adversely affect the child's physical, emotional, psychological or general wellbeing which prevent the enjoyment of his or her rights and who need protection" (National Policy on Orphans and Vulnerable Children, 2009, p. 5). In Botswana children are considered vulnerable based on several needs and it depends from one group to the other. The following children are considered vulnerable: street children, child laborers, children who are sexually exploited, neglected children, those with disability, and those living in remote areas forming part of the minority groups (Skinner et al., 2006). Also, a vulnerable child refers to someone who has no, or limited, access to basic needs and whose rights are denied even if they live with both parents (Skinner et al., 2004).

The Situation of HIV/AIDS

Botswana is one of the hardest hit countries by the HIV and AIDS pandemic in sub-Saharan Africa. With its population of about two million (Central Statistics Office, 2001; Ministry of Health, 2009), its HIV prevalence rate for the general population was estimated at 17.6 percent in 2008 and now stands at 18.5 percent (Central Statistics Office, 2009; Republic of Botswana, 2013). The age-specific prevalence rates in 2008 were as follows: 1.5–4 years (2.2 percent), 5–9 years (4.7 percent), 10–14 years (3.5 percent), and 15–19 years (3.7 percent) (Central Statistics Office, 2009). This prevalence among young children is an indication of transmission of the HIV from mother to child. The general population prevalence rate suggests that more females (19.2 percent) than males (14.1 percent) are infected with HIV. The observed gender disparity may be explained by men's dominance in sexuality matters as encouraged by the Setswana culture and socio-economic differences—as noted, women, especially single women, are likely to live under the poverty datum line. Due mainly to the high prevalence rate among adults, the country has a large number of orphaned children (Department of Social Services, 2008; UNICEF/UNAIDS, 2009). In 2007, 6.5 percent of all children had lost both parents while 17.2 percent of all children had lost at least one parent (Department of Social Services, 2010; Ministry of Health, 2009). The impact of HIV and AIDS coupled with poverty has created high levels of vulnerability among children. A significant proportion of these receive protection and support, mainly through foster care. Indeed, data from the Department of Social Services (2006) suggest that about 95 percent of orphans in the country are absorbed within the kinship systems of care. Given the significance of foster care in the welfare of children made vulnerable by HIV/AIDS, below we provide an overview of the practice of fostering in Botswana.

The Practice of Fostering in Botswana

Fostering is the practice of allowing children to be reared by people other than their biological parents (McDaniel and Zulu, 1996). It is a way of providing a stable family life for children and young people who are unable to live with their parents. This allows them the chance to thrive in a safe, secure, loving, and caring home environment. In the context of most sub-Saharan African countries, formal foster care is not a common approach; instead, children in need of care live in informal foster or customary care arrangements. This kind of fostering stems from customs whose origins are deeply embedded in African cultures (Goody, 1982). In varying degrees, kin provide shelter, emotional support, educational support, material support, spiritual support as well as moral support to children in need of care. According to the Department of Social Services (2006), at least 95 percent of orphans in the country are absorbed within the kinship structures based on descent and marriage. Like in many African countries, kinship care is not regulated by formal institutions or laws. Therefore, human service professionals such as social workers rarely intervene in the placement of children in kinship care because of the authoritative roles that relatives play in such placements. As suggested in the foregoing overview, there are two major types of foster care systems in Botswana. These are kinship/customary care and statutory foster care. An overview of these systems is provided in this section.

Customary Care

Customary care has been part of the Tswana culture. The extended family has traditionally played an important role in caring for children who could not live with their biological parents for one reason or another. From time immemorial, the extended family, in Botswana, has been known for its role of caring for and supporting orphans and other members in need of assistance. Customary foster care enables children to grow up as part of the family and community, with a sense of identity and belonging (Tsheko et al., 2007a).

Traditionally, caring and nurturing included both material support and use of story-telling by elders to help children cope with the death of their parents. Today, the tradition of fostering by the extended family has continued and is an important coping mechanism in countries like Botswana, which have experienced high HIV prevalence and growing orphan populations (Miller et al., 2006). This practice exists on a large scale because it flows naturally from traditional values, practices, and societal expectations on the extended family system to care for and protect disadvantaged members. The government of Botswana's position on the practice is that children classified as vulnerable are better served when cared for by the extended family and communities rather than by non-relatives. Moreover, from a family preservation perspective, the extended family is seen as an important transmitter of cultural capital, an essential element in the growth and development of the child. Furthermore, kinship systems emphasize sibling bonds, providing a sense of belonging and security to children. There is also some evidence to suggest that when children are placed with people they know (Testa and Rolock, 1999), they tend to report better outcomes. They also have the benefit of living and growing up in their communities. This has the potential to strengthen the child's sense of identity and self-esteem. It also highlights a communal responsibility for the wellbeing of children. Another advantage of fostering by the extended family is that the extended family is seen as culturally acceptable and assumed to be sustainable through a child's development (Deininger et al., 2003). Further, as observed by Tshitswana (2003), the extended family has been the traditional social security system; providing protection to the vulnerable, care for those who were sick and poor, and transmission of social values and education to children. Indeed, despite resource and financial constraints, the extended family continues to be the most effective safety net for children classified as vulnerable in Botswana (Madhavan, 2004). Currently, an estimated 90 percent of orphaned children live in households with extended family members including aunts, uncles, grandparents, and other relatives serving as primary caregivers (Miller, 2006).

Although the extended family continues to be a sound source of stability, love, and emotional care for children classified as vulnerable, problems abound within the kinship system. First, the extended family has been stretched beyond its capacity and in many instances has lost the ability to provide care. In addition, the current settlement patterns (rural versus urban) present a challenge. With urbanization and industrialization, people are mobile, moving from rural to urban areas. Consequently, this has impacted both the quantity and quality of mutual support that relatives could provide in time of need. Furthermore, research evidence suggests that children who are taken in by the extended family are likely to be mistreated, abused, and exploited (Foster, 2004). This is often the case with girls, who may experience sexual exploitation at the hand of caregivers charged with the responsibility of protecting them. In addition, caregivers are known to burden orphaned children with domestic chores, infringing on their right to leisure and education.

Statutory Foster Care

Although provisions for statutory foster care are in place, currently, the country does not have a national formal foster care program. As is the case in many countries of sub-Saharan Africa, this type of foster care does not exists on a large scale and is provided through residential care facilities for Orphans and Vulnerable Children (OVC). In 2008, for example, between 500 and 600 children were housed in all the residential care facilities in the country (Maundeni, 2009). Statutory care (in the form of residential care) to OVC in Botswana is offered by four institutions. These are Childline Botswana, Save Our Souls (SOS), Mpule Kwelagobe Centre, and Paolo Zanichelli Children's Home (USAID, 2010). A brief description of these is provided below. These organizations aim to protect vulnerable children on a short-, medium-, and/or long-term basis. They provide safe environments that respect the rights of children. Services offered at these institutions include: temporary and permanent shelter, food and clothing, counseling, healthcare, and training and education on a short- or long-term basis.

Placement of children under statutory care is a multi-faceted process which begins with identification of children considered OVC. Identification is often carried out by community members including chiefs, headmen, and village child-welfare committee members, as well as by service providers such as family welfare educators and community health nurses. Selected children are then referred to social workers. At school they are identified by the teachers in collaboration with the Parent Teacher Organization (PTA). It should be noted at this juncture that, according to the Botswana Children's Act of 2009, each village is mandated to have a village child protection committee (VCPC), which comprises, among others, the chief and the social worker as ex-officio members. The chief in the context of Botswana is a person who is well respected by his community. The fact that the Act makes it mandatory for chiefs to sit in VCPCs shows that the country takes child welfare issues seriously. To some extent it also makes chiefs to be invested in, and sensitive to child welfare issues within their communities.

Residential care facilities for children classified as OVC in Botswana are structured into family units to reflect the family structure in Botswana. Siblings are usually placed in the same family unit. Below we provide a brief description of these. Below we give a brief description of organizations that include shelter in their services.

Save Our Souls Children's Villages

Save Our Souls Children's Villages is a private child welfare organization whose aim is to provide a home and family for destitute, abandoned, and orphaned children. It offers residential care and has adopted a family model where children are grouped in smaller family units headed by SOS "mothers" (Alao and Molojwane, 2008). For instance, a typical SOS facility will consist of 10–15 houses/units each led by a SOS mother. Each unit holds 6–10 children (either boys or girls) who stay as brothers and sisters, headed by a caregiver charged with the responsibility of providing care to the children in that particular unit (Maundeni, 2009; USAID, 2010). The facility strives to develop children into responsible adults, capable of living independent lives outside the Village.

Childline Botswana

Childline Botswana is a non-governmental organization (NGO) founded in 1990 in response to the escalating number of child abuse cases in the country. Its primary mission is to help abused children and address other child welfare related issues through nurturing and strategies such as the provision of accommodation, education, counseling, and an alternative care program. The agency offers temporary emergency accommodation and care for up to 20 children below the age of five years. Childline Botswana sees institutionalization of children as an option to be utilized only when a child cannot be placed in a family environment. Childline Botswana has also collaborated with the Department of Social Service (DSS) in promoting foster care programs in the country.

Mpule Kwelagobe Centre

This center started operating in 2000 with the goal of providing accommodation to abused and orphaned children (UNICEF, 2007). The services offered by Mpule Kwelagobe Children's Village in Botswana include shelter, counseling, and medical attention to children affected by and infected with HIV.

The Paolo Zanichelli Children's Home

The goals of this Kalahari children's home is to raise children in a safe and calm environment where they will be cared for, nurtured, and loved. Services provided include education and healthcare. The goal is to create a safe haven—a big family—where the children will be educated and learn values including fraternity, solidarity, and independence.

Different professionals are employed in residential care centers to attend to the various needs of the children. However, for the purpose of this chapter, the role of only two professionals will be highlighted: nurses and social workers.

Nurses in the Foster Care System

Nurses are employed to provide holistic and continued care to ensure a comprehensive and coordinated treatment approach by all professionals involved in the care of children. The OVC require initial health screenings and comprehensive assessment for their medical, mental, dental, and developmental status (UNICEF and Botswana University, 2010). It should be noted that some fostered children get admitted as newborn infants and young children. These infants are immediately taken to the hospitals where they remain until referred to residential care facilities or are adopted. Those in foster institutions need to be followed up by nurses and midwives to monitor their growth and development as well as to administer immunizations according to the Expanded Programme on Immunization (EPI).

Children in foster care are prone to chronic and complex illnesses as compared to those in normal environment. They may be HIV positive and prone to opportunistic infections. Children affected by or infected with HIV need special support to cope with the burden of illness and/or death in their families. The nurse equips caretakers with the necessary knowledge and skills to care for children in foster institutions. Some OVC are living with HIV and AIDS and are on antiretroviral drugs (ARVs). The nurse has to ensure that the OVC adhere to medications and protect them from stigma and discrimination. Therefore assessing each child's unique needs is critical (UNICEF and Botswana University, 2010). The nurse in the center provides guidance to the caregivers with regard to the children's healthcare management. These children require thorough assessment by a nurse because information received about their health status before placement is often missing or hard to obtain. Therefore, the major roles and responsibilities of nurses are as follows:

- initial health screening and provision of emergency care to abandoned infants and babies;
- comprehensive health assessment of all OVC prior to placement in foster care settings;
- provision and continuity of primary care and monitoring of health status in foster homes/institutions;
- evaluation of developmental and mental health status (UNICEF and Botswana University, 2010).

Social Workers in the Foster Care System

Social workers employed in residential care facilities for OVC in Botswana provide psychosocial support. Some of the children placed in care have experienced prolonged trauma, therefore intense efforts need to be made to rehabilitate them and their families. Social workers also ensure that children in care get protection against all forms of abuse and enjoy their rights. In some cases when children are admitted to the facilities, they may have already experienced traumatic events that may jeopardize their wellbeing. As such, some attention is given to preventing children's exposure to additional trauma as well as psychosocial rehabilitation. The children also work closely with social workers employed in other organizations to rehabilitate the children's families of origin in preparation for when the children exit care institutions and are placed with these families.

Social workers who work in residential care facilities also work hand-in-hand with counterparts who are employed in organizations, such as: policy formulation and advocacy; sensitization of communities about issues which adversely affect children's wellbeing such as child abuse, family violence, orphanhood as well as HIV/AIDS; property grabbing; children's rights; child abuse; and peer pressure. They also distribute Information Education and Communication (IEC) material on such issues. Some social workers participate in radio and TV discussions that focus on these issues. Other roles that social workers play include education and training (preventive work), for example, Childline Botswana has modules that focus on child abuse, children's rights, disciplining children, children and feelings, and children and trauma. In recent years, social workers working for Childline Botswana have also been training potential foster parents on foster care.

The Cost of Fostering

Support for the running of the residential care facilities comes from the government of Botswana and NGOs. According to USAID (2010), the government spends a total of BPW 54,666,788 (US$7,822,817) on OVC services each year. BPW 7,292,320 (US$1,043,531) is spent by the government on shelter and care alone; this sum accounts for about 13 percent of total spending on OVC care (USAID, 2010). Overall, the money provided for OVC care is not enough. Indeed, many NGOs operate under financial constraints. The situation has been exacerbated by the fact that most international donor agencies have reduced their funding to Botswana under the contention that they prefer to channel funds to more needy countries (Moatshe, 2004).

Who are the Children Living in Foster Care Arrangements in Botswana?

Before describing the characteristics of children living in foster care arrangements in Botswana, it is important to reiterate that, in the absence of biological parents and declining capacity of the extended family to care for children classified as vulnerable, a considerable proportion continues to be pushed in statutory care although informal foster care is desirable. The country does not have a large scale formal foster care system despite attempts to introduce one. Reasons for the failure of the proposed national foster care program include the principle that foster parents were not to receive compensation or remuneration from the government (Dahl, 2012). Another reason for the popularity of informal foster care/customary care is that formal adoption in Botswana is uncommon. It is important to note that the traditional system of care characterized by placing children within the extended family is popular as it allows for continuity and transmission of traditional values and practices.

Children living in foster care arrangements in Botswana are diverse. They vary in terms of age, gender, family, socio-economic background, and other characteristics. Orphans are highly represented among children in informal foster care. With the advent of HIV and AIDS, Botswana has seen the death of many parents. Orphans are fostered because of the absence of biological parents. Other children are placed in foster care because they may have experienced abandonment, neglect, extreme poverty, mental illness, homelessness, HIV infection, and sexual abuse, especially by close relatives (Seboni, 2010; Tsheko et al., 2007b; Maundeni, 2009). Another group of children likely to be found in foster care are children whose parents tend to move from one place to another. As noted, many people in the country tend to move seasonally. For instance, during the ploughing season, adults tend to spend most of the time in the farms while in the period immediately after the rainy season, women go out for days to cut thatch or collect *mophane* worms. Oftentimes, it is not convenient to take young children with them. Such children are temporarily left in the care of the extended family members, with the parent resuming full care of their children upon return. This is usually short-term and not considered fostering in the context of Batswana culture. The third group of children found in foster care is children from poor homes. It is not uncommon for poor single mothers who work in low-paying jobs in towns to leave their children with relatives in rural areas. In contrast, people who live in rural areas believe that their children will have a better start in life if they live with relatives in the urban areas, where access to education and health facilities are better. For large families, both in the urban and rural areas, the pressure of looking after children can be overwhelming both financially and physically, and the option of sending children to live with relative is utilized when it is available. Better-off family members often come to the aid of their relatives by agreeing to take over the care of children when family resources are strained.

Experiences of Fostered Children in Botswana

Existing literature shows that fostered children have diverse experiences (Thamaku and Daniel, 2013; Ngwenya and Phaladze, 2007; UNICEF, 2002; Lindsey et al., 2003; Raditedu, 2004). These include both positive and negative ones. Positive experiences consist of perceived social support, being cared for, going to school, participating in school and other community activities, making friends, and having role models (Seboni, 2010). In fact, even deceased parents were identified as role models. Similar sentiments have been reported by respondents in a recent study (Thupayagale-Tshweneagae et al., 2005), who pointed out that being fostered allowed them to receive support from close relatives, service providers (nurses, doctors, and social workers), their guardians in foster homes, teachers, and from their friends. They indicated that their relatives accompanied them to follow-up care. In addition to this, the opportunity enabled them to attend school. Like other adolescents, the children demonstrated a sound future orientation and emphasized the importance of having a career and a job. In fact, most of them have set some long-term goals. These were predominantly based on good performance at school and having a career, getting married, and having children.

Negative experiences of fostered children consist of exposure to stigma and discrimination, abuse, neglect, movement of orphans from one relative to another, separation of siblings as a result of placement in different homes for economic reasons, and property grabbing (see UNICEF, 2002; Lindsey et al., 2003; Tsheko et al., 2007b; Maundeni and Malinga-Musamba, 2013). Tsheko and colleagues have noted that some caregivers use fostered children for their own economic gains. They asserted that relatives from poor families sometimes fight over the custody of orphaned children in order to benefit from government services for OVC, such as food baskets and clothing. The above-mentioned negative experiences adversely affect the children's wellbeing. Furthermore, a study by Tsheko et al. (2007b) on OVC revealed that they were unhappy with the lack of support and care received from their guardians.

Social Benefits Associated with Fostering

The benefits of foster care for children classified as OVC include, among others, provision of food and nutrition, counseling, clothing and bedding, shelter, adult supervision/protection as well as social support. Another benefit is intergenerational transfer of intellectual and life skills. Further, as observed by Testa and Rolock (1999), when OVC are placed with the extended families, they experience reduced depression and isolation, as well as separation from one's culture and community. In a sense, therefore, psychosocial wellbeing may be an important outcome of fostering.

At the societal level, benefits may consist of community cohesion, a positive externality attributed to the feeling of togetherness experienced by community members united around the goal of supporting children who have lost their biological parents (Deininger et al., 2003). Other gains that may be accrued to society include provision of safe and nurturing environment for children. This has the potential to create long-term effects such as cultural preservation, national development, increased productivity, and reduced crime.

Challenges of Foster Care in Botswana

There are several challenges inherent in both customary and statutory practices of fostering. These are experienced by the OVC, their foster families and institutions as well as the service providers. One of the challenges in both customary care and formal care is inadequate attention paid to children's psychosocial issues. According to Thamuku and Daniel (2013), most programs for orphans in the country provide tangible forms of assistance, giving little attention to grief counseling and other psychosocial needs.

Moreover, family members have a tendency to make decisions for the OVC regarding their future, their property, and living arrangements. Since members of the extended family often have their own children, it is not uncommon for orphan-siblings to be shared by members of the extended family, thus separating them from one another. The sharing is mainly for economic reasons, however, it may complicate the orphans' adjustment to parental loss.

Another challenge that is hardly documented is the culture of silence surrounding issues related to HIV and death (Thamuku and Daniel, 2013). A majority of children who participated in Thamuku and Daniel's study indicated that they had not discussed the experience of loss with anyone before their participation in therapy. They associated their reluctance to talk about death-related issues with anyone with fear—fear of the dead, of being ridiculed by adults, of excessive pain that could awaken when attempting to address the issue of marginalization, and of hurting the deceased parent. The culture of silence surrounding death also stems from the beliefs that children need protection from harsh realities (van der Heijden and Swartz, 2010). Examples from study participants include:

> At home, I have been told that talking about death brings bad luck to the family. I don't want my mother to torture me. [Female participant]

Another had this to say:

> I told my aunt how my mama's death has really hurt me ... She cried too and said we better not talk about it. She said it can be scary. She gave me money for sweets and asked me to go and play.

Another challenge is the lack of information children are given on HIV, the status of family members, and their own status. Respondents in a study conducted by Thupayagale-Tshweneagae et al. (2005) revealed that their HIV positive status was not disclosed to them until the age of 13 and 14 years, even though they were often sick most of their lives. This feeds directly into the culture of silence alluded to in the foregoing discussion.

The continued rise in the numbers of children who need foster care is another challenge. Unfortunately, available figures on the phenomenon are not reliable as many cases go unreported. Recent increases in cases of abandoned children may be an indication that many families are unable to take care of their children, suggesting the need to expand residential homes for such children.

Another side to this story relates to problems experienced by caregivers. These consist of financial, health, and emotional issues. Indeed, the majority of caregivers in the country are elderly women (see Maundeni and Malinga-Musamba, 2013, for a detailed discussion of these problems). Other challenges faced by caregivers in Botswana include the following: limited information about orphan care programs (Ngwenya and Phaladze, 2007), inadequate parenting skills, lack of support from other relatives (Hlabyago and Ogunbanjo, 2009), conflicts among caregivers and other relatives, inadequate attention to caregivers' needs, and limited preparation for the caregiving role. Daniel (2003) also argues that in many poor households where there are no alternative sources of income, orphans have become breadwinners because of their monthly food basket from the government. Caregivers therefore feel that this has the potential to negatively influence the behavior of dependent adolescents—they may become proud, arrogant, and sometimes disrespectful.

Statutory foster care has its own unique challenges, paramount among these is the high cost associated with operations and overheads. Other costs include determining management eligibility and ongoing facility monitoring. According to Tsheko (2007), statutory foster care costs up to 10 times more than care within a family unit. Moreover, some children tend to stay in the facilities longer than intended when they were placed (Maundeni, 2009). The observed trends are not only peculiar to Botswana, they are well documented in existing literature from other countries (cf. Sinclair and Gibbs, 1998).

Reflection on How to Address Challenges in the Foster Care System

The foregoing discussion reveals that informal foster care is the common form of care in Botswana, with the extended family playing a major role. A small percentage of children are housed in formal residential care facilities. It has also shown that several challenges exist in the foster care system of Botswana. These include: limited involvement of OVC in the decisions that affect them, and inadequate attention to psychosocial support as well as an increase in the number of abandoned children. Caregivers also present challenges including poor health, poverty, and lack of parenting skills. The main dilemma faced by residential care facilities is the high cost of running them in an era of economic recession. In this section, we attempt to provide our views on how some of these issues could be addressed in order to improve the experiences of children classified as "vulnerable."

Some of the ways to address challenges in the foster care system include expanding and intensifying psychosocial support programs for fostered children, as well as empowering caregivers to better meet the unique and multi-faceted needs of OVC. Developing a national foster care program may be important in this regard. The socio-economic conditions of orphans and vulnerable children may require some attention. Indeed, studies have shown that one of the major problems experienced by children defined as vulnerable is poverty—caregivers, mostly maternal grandmothers, survive on destitute rations and old age pensions (initially P110, now P220 [approximately U$19 and U$36.7, respectively]). Adequate material and psychosocial support may need to be provided to such families. In addition, effort could be made to place siblings in the same home.

There is also the issue of baby/child abandonment. One way of addressing this might be enactment of a safe haven law making provision for the following: (1) allowing an individual to safely and anonymously place a baby at a designated location without fear of being arrested; (2) empowering the safe haven to provide basic services to the child; and (3) sensitizing both males and females about the dangers of unplanned pregnancies as well as the responsibility for their children, whether they are born within marriage or out of wedlock. Since the majority of orphans have lost parents as a result of HIV and AIDS, services provided by the safe haven may involve assessment of the child's HIV status in order to facilitate timely provision of the necessary services such as ARVs.

The culture of silence surrounding death may need to be addressed as a matter of urgency. For the most part, orphaned children are rarely engaged in discussions about how they are coping with the death of their parents. Further, other emotional needs they may present are rarely taken into account. Generally, there is a shortage of programs that provide psychosocial support to OVC, suggesting the need to develop these. A model that may be explored is the group approach that uses peers to provide psychosocial support to bereaved children. At the time of writing this chapter, one such program—EARTH therapy (an intervention which aims to strengthen orphans' capacity to be well-functioning young adults)—has been adopted by the government of Botswana and is being scaled up across 10 out of 16 districts (Kvissellien, 2012; Thamuku and Daniel, 2013).

Although customary foster care is the cheapest and most common living arrangement for OVC, there is a need to increase the number of foster care institutions to keep up with the growing number of OVC in the country. This could reduce the length of time abandoned children stay in hospitals as they await placement. In addition, attention could focus on supporting school-age OVC to complete their education and acquire skills that will enable them to become responsible adults who contribute meaningfully to their communities and the welfare of the nation. It is common knowledge that children classified as OVC suffer abuse and exploitation, even when cared for by relatives. Mechanisms to protect OVC from abuse and exploitation need to be put in place and strengthened where they already exist.

Finally, Botswana is a signatory to the Convention on the Rights of Child (CRC) and has domesticated its requirements in national laws; enforcement of some of the clauses, however, still lags behind. The CRC purports that the child's evolving capacity needs to be recognized and respected, so that they can be involved in decisions that will impact their future. Children classified as OVC have not been involved in the decision-making process even when these decisions directly affect their welfare. This may be because the country lacks mechanism for monitoring and reinforcement of policy decisions. The reality for OVC has been exploitation and the infringement of their rights. The parties concerned, including the government of Botswana, may need to revisit this issue with the goal of addressing gaps in implementation and enforcement of CRC requirements.

Conclusion

This chapter has examined the nature of fostering in Botswana, experiences of fostered children, benefits of fostering, challenges in the foster care system, as well as solutions to address these challenges. It is clear that customary foster care is the most common and desirable type of care provided to OVC in Botswana. Customary fostering is important in promoting the spirit of self-reliance and family preservation. It is also looked at as an expression of a compassionate nation that protects and cares for its own, especially the vulnerable. However, against the backdrop of the ongoing scourge of HIV and AIDs, customary fostering can only remain a viable option with the relevant policies and programs in place. Members of the extended family who care for OVC need to be supported both financially and socially by the government, the private sector, and the business community. At the same time, given the increasing trend in child abandonment, it is necessary to further develop and strengthen foster care institutions, even as a temporary measure. For both customary and institution-based fostering, a key issue is child-centered psychosocial support to heal the emotional pain of OVC, and to provide a platform for healthy growth and development. Finally, within the entirety of the fostering system, the rights of fostered children need to be recognized and upheld so that the vulnerable of today can become tomorrow's productive and responsible citizens.

Bibliography

Alao, A.A. and Molojwane, M.B. (2008). Childhood sexual abuse: The Botswana perspective. In Smith, M.J. (ed.), *Child Sexual Abuse: Issues and Challenges*. New York: Nova Science Publishers.

Central Statistics Office (2001). *Botswana AIDS Impact Survey*. Gaborone, Botswana: Author.

Central Statistics Office (2005). *Botswana AIDS Impact Survey II 2004 Statistical Report*. Gaborone, Botswana: Author.

Central Statistics Office (2009). *Botswana AIDS Impact Survey III 2008 Statistical Report*. Gaborone, Botswana: Author.

Central Statistics Office (2013). *Botswana AIDS Impact Survey 2012 Statistical Report*. Gaborone, Botswana: Author.

Committee on Early Childhood, Adoption and Dependent Care (2002). Health care of young children in foster care. *American Academy of Paediatrics*, 109–536.

Dahl, B. (2010). Failed Fostered: Concepts of Family and Care Giving in Botswana 'Unsuccessful' Formal Foster Care Program for Orphans. Brown University. http://paa2010.princeton.edu/papers/101855.

Dahl, B. (2012). An Anthropological Demographic Evaluation of Why Botswana's National Formal Foster Care Program for Orphans Failed. http://uaps2011.princeton.edu/papers/110989.

Daniel, M. (2003). Listening to orphan voices. In Biakolo, E., Mathangwane, J. and Odallo, D. (eds), *The Discourse of HIV/AIDS in Africa* (pp. 117–19). UNAIDS, ICT, Pretoria.

Deininger, K., Jin, S., Adenew, B., et al. (2003). Tenure security and land-related investment: evidence from Ethiopia. Policy Research Paper 2991. Washington, DC, World Bank.

Department of Social Services (2006). *A Report on Provision of Psychosocial Services to Orphans and Vulnerable Children in Botswana: Issues and Challenges*. Ministry of Local Government, DSS.

Department of Social Services (2008). *National Guidelines on the Care of Orphans and Vulnerable Children*. Ministry of Local Government, DSS.

Department of Social Services (2010). *Botswana National Plan of Action for Orphans and Vulnerable Children, 2010–2016*. Gaborone, Botswana: Author.

Foster, G. (2004). Safety nets for children affected by HIV/AIDS in Southern Africa. In Foster, G. and Pharoah, R. (eds), *A Generation at Risk: HIV/AIDS, Vulnerable Children and Security in Southern Africa* (pp. 65–92). Cape Town, South Africa: Institute of Security Studies.

Goody, E.N. (1982). *Parenthood and Social Reproduction: Fostering and Occupational Roles in West Africa*. Cambridge: Cambridge University Press.

Government of Botswana (1999). *Short-term Plan of Action for the Care of Orphans in Botswana*. Gaborone, Botswana: Ministry of Local Government.

Government of Botswana (2008). *National Guidelines on the Care of Orphans and Vulnerable Children*. Gaborone, Botswana: Ministry of Local Government, Department of Social Services.

Government of Botswana (2008a). *National Situation Analysis on Orphans and Vulnerable Children in Botswana*. Gaborone, Botswana: Ministry of Local Government, Department of Social Services.

Government of Botswana (2009). *Children's Act*. Gaborone, Botswana: Parliament of Botswana.

Hlabyago, K.E. and Ogunbanjo, G.A. (2009). The experiences of family caregivers concerning their care of HIV/AIDS orphans. *South African Family Practice*, 51(6), 506–11.

Kvissellien, I.M. (2012). Thriving in a time of transition: Orphaned youth in Lothlakane East, Botswana (Electronic Thesis or Dissertation). https://bora.uib.no/bitstream/handle/1956/5877/94439165.pdf?sequence=1.

Lindsey, E.L., Hirschfeld, M., Tlou, S., and Ncube, E. (2003). Home-based care in Botswana: Experiences of older women and young girls. *Health Care for Women International*, 24, 486–501.

Madhavan S. (2004). Fosterage patterns in the age of AIDS: Continuity and change. *Social Science and Medicine*, 58(7), 1443–54.

Maundeni, T. (2009). Residential care for children in Botswana: The past, the present, and the future. In Courtney, M.E. and Iwaniec, D. (eds), *Residential Care for Children: Comparative Perspectives* (pp. 88–105). New York: Oxford University Press.

Maundeni, T. and Malinga-Musamba, T. (2013). The role of informal caregivers in the wellbeing of orphans in Botswana: A literature review. *Child and Family Social Work*, 18, 107–16.

McDaniel, A. and Zulu, E. (1996). Mothers, fathers, and children: Regional patterns in parent-child residence in sub-Saharan Africa. *Etudes de la Population Africaine*, 11, 28–9.

Miller, C.M., Gruskin, S., Subramanian, S.V., et al. (2006). Orphan Care in Botswana's Working Households: Growing Responsibilities in the Absence of Adequate Support. *American Journal of Public Health*, 96(8), 1429–35.

Ministry of Health (2009). *Accelerated Child Survival and Development Strategy 2009/10–2015/16*. Gaborone, Botswana: Author.

Ministry of Local Government, Housing and Lands (1999). *Short Term Plan of Action for the Care of Orphans*. Department of Social Services, Gaborone.

Moatshe, B. (2004). The Impact of Declining Donor Support on the Sustainability of Non-Governmental Organizations in Botswana: Insights from Some NGO Managers in Botswana (unpublished Bachelor of Social Work dissertation). Department of Social Work, University of Botswana.

National Policy on Orphans and Vulnerable Children (2009). http://www.gov.bw/tn/Search-Results/?quicksearchquery=national+policy+on+orphans+and+vulnerable+children&lan=tn-ZA.

Ngwenya, B.N. and Phaladze, N.A. (2007). Access to support and human rights—challenges for older carers of orphaned children in Botswana. In Jacques, G., Lesetedi, G. and Osei-Hwedie, K. (eds), *Human Rights and Social Development in Southern Africa* (pp. 213–34). Gaborone: Bay Publishing.

Phaladze, N., Seboni, N.M., and Seloilwe, E.S. (2009). Adherence to ARVs by adolescents living with HIV and AIDS. The National HIV and AIDS conference held in Gaborone in 1998 Project Concern International. http://www.projectconcern.org/site.

Raditedu, B.L. (2004). Psychosocial Impact of Orphan Hood on the Girl-Child: A Study of Kalkfotein (unpublished Bachelor of Social Work dissertation). Department of Social Work, University of Botswana.

Republic of Botswana (2013). Preliminary Results Botswana AIDS Impact Survey IV. Stats Brief 2013(28). Gaborone, Botswana: Statistics Botswana.

Seboni, N.M. (2010). The lived experiences of adolescents living with HIV and AIDS in Botswana. Paper presentation at Tau Lambda Chapter of STTI Conference held in Nairobi, July 30 to August 2, 2010.

Sinclair, I. and Gibbs, I. (1998). *Children's Homes: A Study in Diversity*. New York: John Wiley and Sons.

Skinner, D., Tsheko, N., Mtero-Munyati, S., et al. (2004). *Definition of Orphaned and Vulnerable Children*. Cape Town, South Africa: HSRC.

Skinner, D., Tsheko, N., Mtero-Munyati, S., et al. (2006). Towards a definition of orphaned and vulnerable children. *AIDS Behavior*, 10(6), 619–26.

Sunbeam Fostering Agency (2014). What is fostering? www.sunbeamfostering.com.

Testa, M. and Rolock, N. (1999). Professional foster care: A future worth pursuing? *Child Welfare*, 78(1), 108–24.

Thamuku, M. and Daniel, M. (2013). Exploring responses to transformative group therapy for orphaned children in the context of mass orphaning in Botswana. *Death Studies*, 37(5), 413–47.

Thupayagale-Tshweneagae, G., Seloilwe, E.S., and Dithole, K. (2005). Child fostering in Botswana: A Cultural Perspective. *Pula Botswana Journal of African Studies*, 19(2), 194–200.

Tsheko, G.N. (2007). *Qualitative Research Report on Orphans and Vulnerable Children in Palapye, Botswana.* Cape Town, South Africa: Human Science Research Control.

Tsheko, G.N., Bainame, K., Odirile, L.W., and Segwabe, M. (2007a). *A Baseline Study on Psychosocial Support of Orphans and Vulnerable Children in Two Villages in Botswana.* Cape Town: HSRC Press.

Tsheko, G.N., Segwabe, M.S., Odirile, L.W., and Tlou, S.D. (2007b). Our children our future. From vision to innovative impact. Community responses to orphans and vulnerable children. In Tsheko, G.N. (ed.), *Situational Analysis of the Socio-Economic Conditions of Orphans and Vulnerable Children in Seven Districts in Botswana.* Cape Town: HSRC Press.

Tshitswana, D.S. (2003). Batswana cultural beliefs and practices: Implications for methods of care for AIDS orphans and other vulnerable children in Botswana (Electronic Thesis/Dissertation). https://etd.ohiolink.edu/.

UNAIDS (2009). *AIDS Epidemic Update December 2009.* Geneva.

UNDP (2012). Report on the Regional Dialogue on Women's Political leadership. Nairobi, Kenya: Author. http://www.ke.undp.org/content/dam/kenya/docs/Democratic%20Governance/UNDP%20championing%20womens%20leadership%20booklet3%20(1).pdf.

UNICEF (2007). *The State of the World's Children 2007. Women and Children. The double divided of gender Equality.* New York: Author.

UNICEF and Botswana University (2010). *Thari ya bana. Reflections on Children in Botswana.* The United Nations Children's Fund Botswana Country Office.

UNICEF and Ministry of Local Government (2002). *Situation Analysis on Orphans and Vulnerable Children: Institutional and Community Responses to Orphans and Vulnerable Children in Botswana.* UNICEF and Ministry of Local Government, Gaborone.

UNICEF/UNAIDS (1999). *Children Orphaned by AIDS. Frontline Responses from Eastern and Southern Africa.* New York: UNICEF division of communication.

United Nations General Assembly (1989). *Convention on the Rights of the Child.* Geneva.

USAID (2010). *A Cost Analysis of Selected Orphans and Vulnerable Children (OVC) Programs in Botswana.* USAID/Health Policy Initiative.

Van der Heijden, I. and Swartz, S. (2010). Bereavement, silence and culture within a peer-led HIV/AIDS-prevention strategy for vulnerable children in South Africa. *African Journal of AIDS Research*, 9(1), 41–50.

Chapter 3
Experiences of Children in Residential Care: The Case of Kenya

Protus Lumiti, Alex Ochumbo, and Nicholas Syano

Introduction and Background Information: Country Profile

Kenya lies on the eastern coast of Africa. It is bordered by Somalia, Ethiopia, and Sudan to the north, Tanzania to the south and Uganda to the west. The country covers an area of 580,367 square kilometers. Kenya, a former colony of the British government, gained its independence in 1963. Unlike other countries in sub-Saharan Africa, Kenya has survived nearly five decades as a functioning nation-state, with regular elections, its borders intact and without experiencing protracted conflict.

Kenya is home to a diverse population of about 45 million people, consisting of 42 ethnic groups. Major ethnic groups include the Kikuyu, Luhya, Luo, Kalenjin, Kamba, Masai, and Samburu. The country's official languages are English and Kiswahili (CIA, 2013). Most of the people in this country reside in rural areas—the rate of urbanization is 24 percent with the majority of the urban population living in two primary cities—Nairobi and Mombasa (CIA, 2013). The population of Kenya is relatively young with the majority of people within the 0–24 age range (61.2 percent). The country has a median age of 19.1 years and a life expectancy of 63.5 years. These factors help to explain the country's high youth dependency ration which stands at 76.1 percent (CIA, 2013). They also call attention to both the resources and problems represented within this group.

Kenya is defined as a democratic country with a multiparty political system. The country was a de facto one-party state from 1969 until 1982 when the ruling party made itself the only party in Kenya. In 1991, largely due to pressure for political liberalization, the country adopted a multiparty political system. Generally, elections are held every four years. In recent years, it is worth noting, these elections have been marred by violence and claims of fraud. In 2010, Kenya adopted a new constitution which aims at devolving power to local governments and giving the people of Kenya a stronger voice in decision-making.

Kenya is relatively wealthy and is seen as the most industrialized country in eastern Africa. For years, agriculture has been the backbone of Kenya's economy. Indeed, the country is a primary exporter of products such as coffee, tea, and horticultural products. Other major sources of revenue have been manufacturing and tourism. In fact, tourism has continued to thrive despite threats of terrorism experienced by Kenya and surrounding countries in recent years. As is the case with other countries in the region, international financial lenders and donors continue to be important contributors to the country's economic wellbeing.

Overall, the country has experienced some economic gains over the past few years (IMF, 2014). Indeed, the proportion of people below the poverty line has declined considerably—it stood at 47 percent in 2005–6 and is currently estimated to be about 40 percent (World Bank, 2014; IMF, 2014). It's important to note, however, that systematic assessment of household welfare has not been conducted since 2005. Despite the observed gains, a number of challenges remain. Unemployment is high at around 40 percent. Further, the country has chronic budget deficits and ranks 145th (out of 187 countries) on the United Nations Development Programme's Human Development Index, which measures development in terms of life expectancy, educational attainment, and standard of living (UNDP, 2013). In addition, the maternal mortality ratio, at 488 maternal deaths per 100,000, is among the highest in the region. Furthermore, diseases such as pneumonia, diarrhea, and malaria continue to disproportionately affect children (WHO, 2012). There is also some evidence pointing to economic and social disparities across the country, with the central and western regions reporting poorer outcomes.

Definition of Concepts

Within the context of Kenya, a child is defined as anyone under the age of 18 years (Children's Act, 2001). In fact the age of 18 is the voting age in the country (see Table 3.1 for more definitions). This definition is significant in that Kenya's population is relatively young. As observed earlier, about 50 percent of the country's population is under the age of 18. More specifically, 42.1 percent is below the age of 14 and 18.7 percent below the age of 24 (CIA, 2013). Another factor associated with this is the high youth dependency ration that defines the country (Table 3.1).

The concepts of OVC, as used in Kenya, may also need definition. The term orphan, in Kenya, characterizes a child below the age of 18 whose parent or both parents have died. According to the National Policy on Orphans and Vulnerable Children, the concept includes a child who has lost one or both parents—maternal orphan, parental orphan, double orphan—to HIV and AIDS. It also covers a child or children in need of care and protection (NPAOVC, 2005). Therefore, a child may be perceived as vulnerable on the basis of the child's relationship to HIV and AIDS, caregiver, service provider, gender, stigma, and discrimination among many other factors. Moreover, OVC may include orphaned children and children whose vulnerability results from the parents or caregiver's morbidity, mortality, household poverty or other socio-economic problems that render the child's basic needs unmet. Table 3.2 presents examples of defining characteristics for OVC provided by 23 organizations (service providers) working with children in Kenya.

Table 3.1 Definition of a child in Kenya

Defining category	Age category
Definition of a child	18
Age of majority	18
Minimum age of employment	13
Minimum age of sexual consent	18
Minimum age of marriage	16
Minimum age of criminal responsibility	8
Minimum age of recruitment into the army	18

Note: A child under the age of 18 may be recruited upon the consent of the parents.
Source: Created using data from the African Child Policy Forum (2013, p. 61).

Table 3.2 Defining characteristics for OVC

Organization's definition	Number of organizations
A child who has lost one or both parents to HIV/AIDS	20
A child who has lost one or both parents to other causes	20
A child with at least one parent infected with the HIV virus	18
A child living without adequate adult support	18
A child experiencing abuse	18
A child living on the streets	17
A child in danger of living on the streets	17
A child infected with the HIV virus	17
A stigmatized child	15
A marginalized child	14
A child who is discriminated against	13
Other: Standard definition under the national policy on OVC	2

Source: Created using data from the Center for Global Health and Development (2009, p. 61).

Little attention has been devoted to understanding the magnitude of the OVC problem in Kenya. However, estimates are that about 2.5 million children fall into the category of OVC. Of these, about 54–60 percent are HIV/AIDS related orphans. To fully capture the implications of these figures it is important to understand that over 50 percent of children in Kenya live below the poverty line. Moreover, about 30 percent have stunted growth while 6 percent exhibit signs of wasting. A significant proportion of children in this group live either alone or in female-headed households (11 percent and 24 percent respectively). Furthermore, about 40 percent of these children are likely to reside with their grandparents and 37 percent with relatives (KNBS, 2009).

This review suggests that effort has been undertaken to help understand the characteristics of children in need of assistance. Moreover, attention has been given to ensuring that the categories are broad enough to embrace all children in need of governmental care and protection. The Children Act of 2001 and the 2005 National Policy on Orphans and Vulnerable Children have been utilized as guiding frameworks to ensure adequate coverage. Furthermore the government has created institutions for the rehabilitation and care of children and provides rules and regulations on how to treat children who need special care and protection. Currently, Kenya has an estimated 415 registered charitable institutions working with children (UNCRC, 2004). In this chapter, we provide an overview of one of these institutions: Children of God Relief Institute (COGRI), which consists of two facilities, i.e., Nyumbani Children's Home in Karen, Nairobi and Nyumbani Village in Kitui, Machakos County.

The Situation of HIV/AIDS in Kenya: An Overview

The HIV epidemic in Kenya has evolved since the first case was diagnosed in 1984 and has become one of the major causes of mortality. Through the years, the HIV/AIDS pandemic has placed tremendous burden on the health system, social networks, and the country's economy. Indeed, the epidemic has affected all sectors of society—children, youths, and families. In recent years, data, primarily from Kenya's Demographic and Health Survey (2003, 2008/9) and the AIDS Indicator Survey (KAIS, 2007, 2012) reveal declines in prevalence. Specifically, a decline of about 40 percent has been indicated nation-wide from 1995/6 to 2003. Data also suggests that the prevalence has remained relatively stable during the past 10 years (see Figure 3.1). Although reliable data with respect to HIV prevalence among children is difficult to come by, there is some data suggesting a similar pattern. In particular, in 2003, 20 percent (242,517) of children nation-wide were living with AIDS. Currently, the figure stands at about 190,131 (10 percent) (UNAIDS, 2012; KAIS, 2013). Furthermore, data indicates that about 13,000 children in the 0–14 age category were newly infected with HIV in 2012 (USAID, 2013). The decline in prevalence is noteworthy and is partially attributed to increases in education and awareness, significant behavioral change and rapid scale-up of antiretroviral therapy (ART).

Although the prevalence has taken a downward trend, women continue to be disproportionately affected compared to men (see Table 3.3). The picture holds true especially for younger women (15–24); these tend to report a higher likelihood of being infected by HIV compared to men of the same age. Further, discrepancies exist between rural and urban areas; with urban localities reporting higher levels of infection.

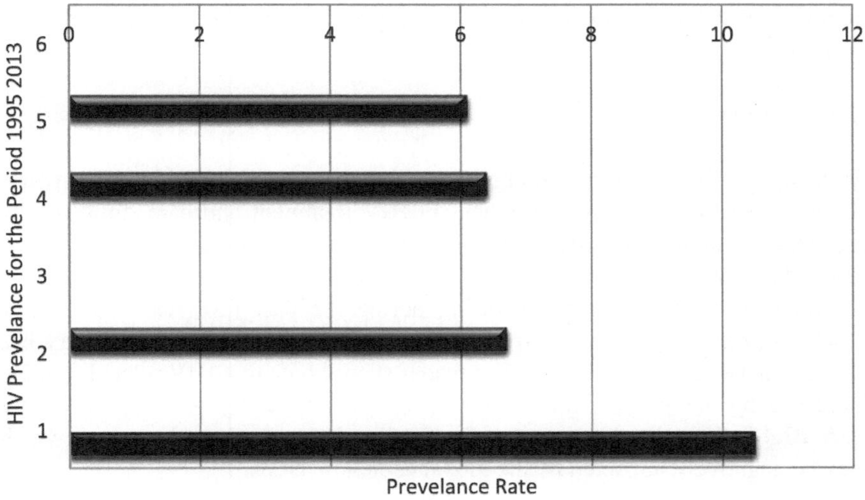

Figure 3.1 Trends in HIV prevalence
Source: Created using data from UNAIDS (2012) and KAIS (2013).

Table 3.3 HIV prevalence among the general population (15–49)

Year	Women	Men
2003	8.9%	4.6%
2008	8.2%	4.3%
2012	6.9%	4.2%

Note: Women in rural areas are more likely to be infected by HIV than men in urban areas (4.5 percent vs. 3.7 percent).
Source: Created using data from KAIS (2013, p. 63).

One of the key effects of the HIV epidemic has been the increased number of children classified as OVC. It is well documented that AIDS related mortality over the years is the primary correlate of the OVC phenomena. Data on OVC is generally not easy to come by. Available data from 2009 to 2013, a period covered in the current national AIDS strategy, indicates a steady decline in the number of AIDS related orphans country-wide: 1,458,103; 1,385,075; 1,307,921; 1,223,377; 1,136,851. These figures, somewhat, contradict projections indicating a steady rise in OVC as the virus continues to claim the lives of people currently living with HIV and AIDS which is estimated at 1.6 million. This may be explained by the fact that the figures alluded to in this discussion reflect reduced mortality due to the ART program. When this is taken into consideration, the projected rise in the number of OVC over time may be significantly high (Center for Global Health and Development, 2009).

Challenges of Note

An analysis of the trend in funding shows that the government of Kenya spends about 50 percent of the total funding on HIV treatment and care, followed by prevention and health system coordination. Overall, only about 9 percent is devoted to OVC care and support.

Kenya has undergone restructuring during the past few years. The effect has been promising on many fronts. However, HIV funding in the country has almost reached its optimal level. The reader should note that HIV related funding increased by about Kshs nine billion over the last five years (approximately US$102,470,760). Further, most of the funding is from external sources, which may be negatively impacted by the global economic crisis.

Fostering in Kenya

As is the case in other parts of Africa, fostering in Kenya generally takes two forms: Formal and informal care. Informal care may be defined as private arrangement provided in a family environment, whereby a non-biological child is looked after on an ongoing basis by the extended family or friends (informal kinship care). This arrangement often lies outside state regulation (Roby and Shaw, 2008). Formal care, on the other hand, is said to be care provided in a family environment which has been ordered/mandated by an administrative body or judicial authority. It also includes care provided in a residential environment, including private facilities. Caregivers are often not related to the child in any way (see Figure 3.2).

In subsequent sections, we highlight the extended family, one of the principal institutions involved in the nurturing and care of children classified as OVC in Kenya. We also present an overview of formal care. The Children of God Relief Institute (COGRI) is used to guide this discussion. This institution was selected because of its leadership in OVC care in the country as well as the innovation of models utilized.

Informal Care

Although faith-based and community organizations continue to be actively engaged in the provision of support to OVC, generally the extended family, friends, and the wider community are the first line of protection and support for children classified as OVC. A number of reasons for this exist. In many parts of Kenya, the extended family is seen as well suited to provide long-term and stable care for a child (International HIV/AIDS Alliance, 2012). The extended family is also believed to

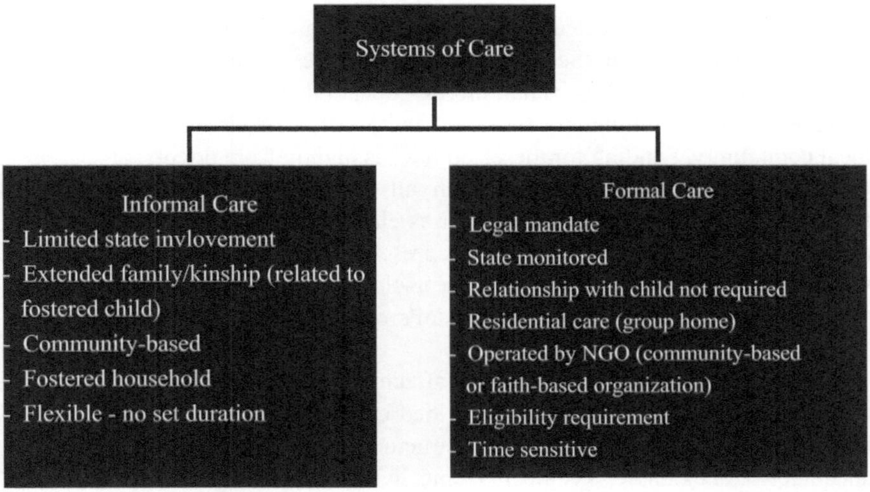

Figure 3.2 Characteristics of foster care
Source: Author.

be a source of nurturing and comfort for a child experiencing the trauma of losing a parent(s). Children also benefit from the emotional support that is provided by the extended family. Given the fact that many families lack the resources to adequately care for OVC, provision of material support to needy families with OVC is seen as a way of ensuring the welfare of such children. For this reason, social protection schemes providing assistance to poorer families have been put in place in areas with high rates of HIV. There is some evidence suggesting that families utilizing social support schemes have experienced a reduction in economic burden (Baird et al., 2013; Haushofer and Shapiro, 2013). Mainly because of these schemes, many children have better nutrition, the opportunity to go to school and better access to healthcare.

Formal Care: The Case of the Children of God Relief Institute (COGRI)

The Children of God Relief Institute (COGRI), popularly known as Nyumbani, was established in 1992. The institute currently operates three facilities: Nyumbani Children's Home in Karen, Nairobi County, Lea Toto and Nyumbani Village in Kitui, Machakos Country. It currently serves about 4,000 children. The institute is dedicated to the promotion of the welfare of orphans who are living with HIV and AIDS.

The institute is guided by the vision of building "Sustainable communities for children infected and affected by the HIV pandemic inspired by Christian compassion." Its primary mission is the provision of quality comprehensive care and support to HIV infected and affected children, families and communities in a sustainable manner. Services provided by the institute include: medical, nutritional, psychosocial, spiritual, moral, educational, and parental care. It also provides a home environment for OVC and assists in their integration into the local community. Funding for these activities is mainly from donors.

Generally, the children come from all over Kenya; Mombasa, Kisumu, Kakamega, Marsabit, Nakuru, Isiolo, or as close as Ngong, Dagoretti, and other areas within and around Nairobi. They represent all ethnicities of Kenya. Children who range in age from newborns to 25-year-olds are referred to Nyumbani through national hospitals and through Nyumbani's own community outreach program, Lea Toto.

Over the years, many infected and affected children and their families have continued to benefit from services provided by the institute. In fact, the institute has diversified its service/intervention structure to meet the needs of the children adequately. For example, Nyumbani Home, in Nairobi, currently cares for 111 HIV positive children; 108 of these are on ARV treatment. There is a lot of improvement in their health. No child died between 2008 and 2010. Further, the home has also established a diagnostic laboratory to serve the children in the programs and the public at large. The home is at the forefront in lobbying for the availability of third-line ARVs in Kenya. The availability of these drugs will reduce mortality rates and enhance the welfare of children living with HIV. A brief overview of the institute's three facilities is provided below.

Nyumbani Children's Home in Karen (Nairobi)

Nyumbani Home was founded to provide holistic care for HIV positive children, who are mostly orphans. The home takes on the structure of a small village/community and is organized in family units. Children are placed in a family unit headed by a house parent—father/mother. At a later stage, the young people are moved to a Youth Centre in preparation for their re-entry into the wider community. It is important to note that the home, through the reintegration program, also traces families and links the young adults to their community. Broadly, while at the home, the children receive life skills training through organized seminars and peer counseling. The goal of these activities is to help the children build self-awareness and self-esteem. In addition to providing a loving home to HIV children and children who have been abandoned, the home also has a respite center and offers nutritional rehabilitation to infants (Figure 3.3 provides the logic model for the home).

The home houses about 120–71 HIV-positive orphans. The age range of residents is from newborns to 23-year-olds. The majority of the children are aged between 13 and 18 years. Indeed, at the moment, the residents consist of 13 toddlers, 70 primary school-age children, 35 teenagers, and 6 young adults (who are in college). The home employs about 50 people. These are responsible for the day-to-day running of the home. Primary activities engaged in cover three broad areas:

1. Holistic family care: Physical, psychosocial, counseling, spiritual and nutritional care.
2. Medical care: Clinical services, laboratory monitoring, nutritional care,
3. Educational: The focus is on encouraging both school attendance and performance. In fact, the home has a pre-school on-site. Older children, for the most part, attend schools within the local community.

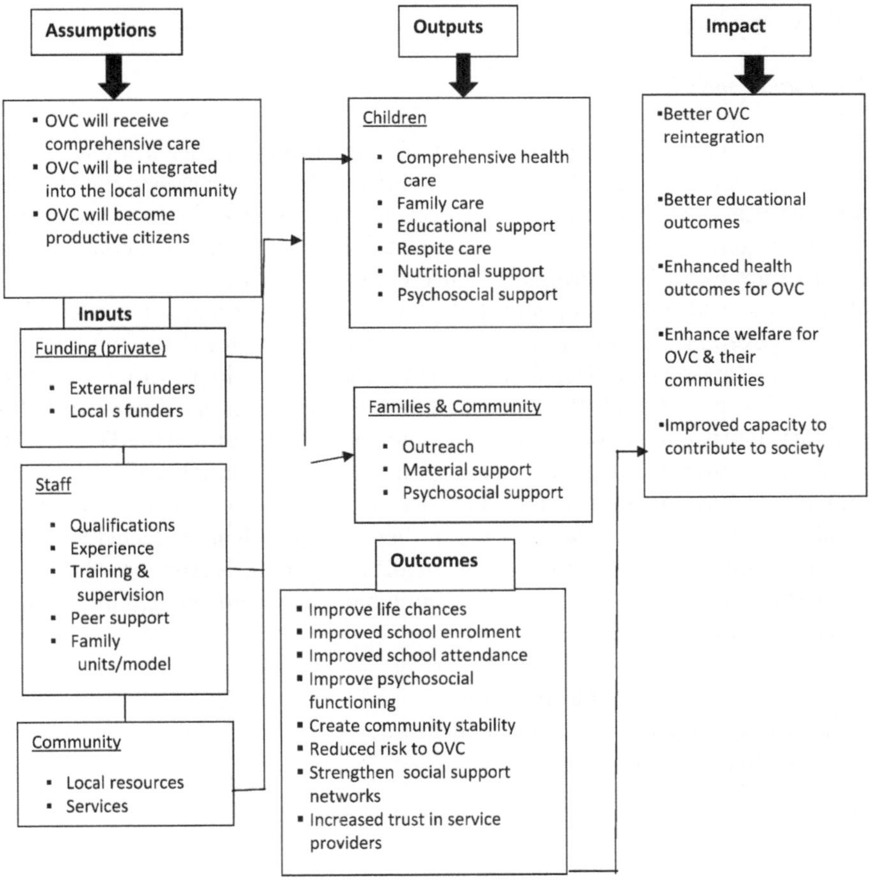

Figure 3.3 Nyumbani Children's Home logic model

Although the impact of the home on the welfare of its young residents has not been systematically evaluated, there is some evidence indicating positive gains. During the past few years, the home has managed to get birth certificates for many of the children in its care. This is a commendable achievement given that most of the children who come to the home are either abandoned or have lost a parent or both parents. In response to the needs arising within the communities served, the home has started a respite center which caters to the needs of critically ill children. Recently, the home has introduced greenhouse farming.

Perhaps the most notable effect is the involvement of the extended family in the lives of children classified as vulnerable who are cared for at the home. The home has launched an initiative to facilitate this. Through this effort, a number of children have been re-integrated with their relatives. Another effect of note is the fact that some children, nurtured through the home, are now gainfully employed and are becoming self-reliant.

Lea Toto Program

Lea Toto is an outreach program of the Children of God Relief Institute which extends Nyumbani's care of HIV positive children into the wider community. The program was established in 1998 and became a fully-fledged community home-based care program a year later. Lea Toto has embraced a partnership model that includes the World Food Program, Concern Worldwide, Medicine for Humanity, Hotcourses, and Kenya Orphanaid. In addition, the organization works with various government ministries. Lea Toto, at the present time, has eight centers: Kangemi, Kawangware, Dagoretti, Kibera, Mukuru, Dandora, Kariobangi, and Mwiki. The program employs about 108 staff and serves an estimated 3,100 children. It sets a target of reaching a cumulative number of 8,500 HIV positive children and over 40,000 family members in Nairobi's informal settlements. The primary objective of the program, which draws its name from Swahili "to raise the child," is improving the quality of life of those living with and affected by HIV/AIDS. To this end, Lea Toto provides medical attention, prevention education, counseling, and life skills, along with community empowerment activities. Other services provided include the following:

1. voluntary counseling and testing;
2. clinical care for home-bound clients;
3. antiretroviral treatment;
4. training of caregivers;
5. nutritional support;
6. micro-credit services to caregivers.

Figure 3.4 provides a brief overview of the program's objectives and impact.

Overall, Lea Toto has affected the lives of served communities positively. Indeed, there is some evidence to suggest that the home-based care and counseling services provided have enabled clients to live more positively. It has also reduced medical-care related spending. One could, therefore, argue that the program is a cost-effective way of meeting the needs of affected individuals and communities.

Despite this observation, challenges remain. Poverty among the people served is relatively high, hence priority is given to basic needs such as food. Another

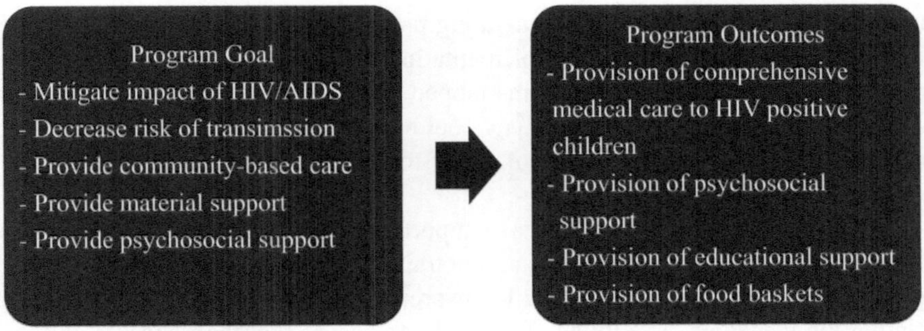

Figure 3.4 Program objectives and impact
Source: Author.

issue relates to social hindrances such as illiteracy, relocation, and caregiver replacement. Further, beliefs and misinformation about HIV and use of ARTs pose as challenges. Coupled with this is the problem of stigma which tends to limit disclosure—negatively impacting adequate support as well as access to services.

Nyumbani Children's Village

Nyumbani Children's Village is situated in Kitui District in the eastern part of Kenya. The organization which was initiated in 2006 is part of the COGRI. It seeks to be a self-sustaining, community-based residential village serving children orphaned as a result of HIV/AIDS. The model utilized involves placing children classified as OVC under the stewardship of an elderly grandparent figure. Unlike traditional orphanages, placing children in family structures ensures nurturing in a home environment, culture transfer, healthcare provision, and high school enrollment and attendance rates.

The concept of Nyumbani Village originated from the need to provide a family atmosphere for OVC under the care of an older relative, most commonly a resource-poor grandmother. Since its inception, the village has only housed one grandfather—who takes care of the children assigned to him single-handedly. In the village, children live together with their guardian as a family unit. Specifically, the families at Nyumbani live in their own houses, till the portion of land allocated to them, and prepare their own meals. Currently, Nyumbani Village is home to 47 grandparents and 443 children. It projects that this will rise to 1,000 children and 250 grandparents in five years. Members of the local community interact with the village on a daily basis. In fact, many of them work as volunteers at the village. The primary objective of the village is to cater to needs of HIV-positive orphans and their caregivers.

Nyumbani Village attempts to promote sustainability and self-reliance. Households at Nyumbani operate on this principle. Hence, the village only provides up to 50 percent of the support needed. To sustain themselves, family units have to engage in income-generating projects and other innovations. Some innovations engaged in include implementation of water conservation and storage technology in the form of sand dams tapped from a seasonal river. The concept of sand dams is relatively new in Kenya but has enormous advantages. The water tapped ensures a constant supply of water for domestic use as well as for drip irrigation purposes.

Services provided include social support, medical and counseling services along with basic education and vocational training. Seminars and peer counseling groups are conducted to help build awareness (HIV/AIDS) and self-esteem among the teenagers. The village also seeks to ensure that the residents and the surrounding communities reach a certain level of self-reliance.

Support for the village comes mainly from external sources including USAID (funding agreement ended in 2012) and other private organizations both within and outside the country.

Although systematic assessment of the program has not been undertaken, there is some evidence indicating that the program has been effective in meeting its objectives. For example, the program has expanded from the two initial grandparents and 19 children to 47 grandparents serving an estimated 443 children. Nearly all the families now have a thriving kitchen garden providing them with vegetables and fruits. Further, the village model has been held as an innovative way of OVC care and is currently replicated in other parts of Africa. A large drip-irrigated farm and livestock unit supplements the families' sustenance. A considerable proportion of land has been planted with trees for both income generation and environmental protection.

Conclusion

Like other countries of the global south, Kenya recorded its first case of HIV in the early 1980s and since then the AIDS epidemic has evolved to become one of the central impediments to national health, wellbeing, and development. It has deepened poverty, slowed economic growth, worsened other infectious diseases, and visited particular ills on affected households, with the harshest effects experienced by women and children. During the past few years, effort has been devoted to the care of OVC. As noted, this has been mainly through the extended family. The Children of God Relief Institute has played a major role in this endeavor. Challenges, however, remain in OVC care. Among these are the magnitude of the problem and the attitude of the general public to the plight of children considered vulnerable. The situation of impoverished children in Kenya is well documented (Ferguson and Heidemann, 2009). A group that has received attention are children who live and work on the streets, who are considered a public nuisance. The entry of OVC on the scene complicates the situation and calls for more comprehensive responses from a broad spectrum of actors.

Another challenge relates to funding and sustainability of current interventions. As noted, HIV funding in the country has almost reached its optimal level. Further, a significant part of these monies are externally sourced. This is unlikely to be sustained overtime. Moreover, OVC care receives only about 9 percent of the total budget of HIV funding.

There is also the issue of monitoring and evaluation of initiatives implemented to address OVC care. In the absence of systematic evaluation, programs continue to be implemented with little empirical guidance. In addition, data gaps continue with regards to the effectiveness of intervention.

Overall, progress has been made in OVC care. The home and village models utilized are promising. Continued effort in the areas of monitoring and evaluation, funding sustainability, and comprehensive care is in need for Kenya, a signatory of the UNAIDS Strategy.

Bibliography

African Child Policy Forum (2013). The African Report on Child Wellbeing – Towards greater accountability to Africa's children. https://app.box.com/s/gnd55soemkrk03wzgqi2/1/1312404009/11737344723/1.

Baird, S., Ferreira, F., Özler, B., and Woolcock, M. (2013). Relative effectiveness of conditional and unconditional cash transfers for schooling in developing countries: A systematic review. *Campbell Systematic Reviews*, 9(8), 1–124.

Central Bureau of Statistics (CBS) [Kenya], Ministry of Health (MOH) [Kenya], and ORC Macro (2004). *Kenya Demographic and Health Survey 2003*. Calverton, Maryland: CBS, MOH, and ORC Macro.

Central Intelligence Agency (2013). The world factbook: Kenya. https://www.cia.gov/library/publications/the-world-factbook/geos/ke.html.

Children's Act (2001). Kenya's Children's Act of 2001. http://www.chr.up.ac.za/undp/domestic/docs/legislation_03.pdf.

Ferguson, K. and Heidemann, G. (2009). Organizational strengths and challenges of Kenyan NGOs serving orphans and vulnerable children: A template analysis. *International Journal of Social Welfare*, 18(4), 354–64.

Haushofer, J. and Shapiro, J. (2013). Policy Brief: Impacts of Unconditional Cash Transfers. http://www.princeton.edu/~joha/publications/Haushofer_Shapiro_Policy_Brief_2013.pdf.

International HIV/AIDS Alliance (2012). *Family-centred HIV Programming for Children: Good Practice Guide*. Hove, UK: Author.

International Monetary Fund (2014). Kenya: Poverty reduction strategy – joint staff advisory note. IMF country report 14/74. http://www.imf.org/external/pubs/ft/scr/2014/cr1474.pdf.

KAIS (2007). Kenya AIDS indicator survey data sheet. Republic of Kenya. http://www.prb.org/pdf09/kaiskenyadatasheet.pdf.

KAIS (2012). Kenya AIDS indicator survey preliminary report. Republic of Kenya. http://nascop.or.ke/library/3d/Preliminary%20Report%20for%20Kenya%20AIDS%20indicator%20survey%202012.pdf.
KAIS (2013). Final report. http://www.faces-kenya.org/wp-content/uploads/2013/09/THE-FINAL-COUNTY-PROFILES-REPORT-FOR-KENYA-revised_2.pdf.
Kenya AIDS epidemic update, The (2012).
Kenya at the United Nations (n.d.). The permanent mission of the Republic of Kenya at the United Nations: General information about Kenya. http://www.kenyaun.org/AboutKenya.aspx?AspxAutoDetectCookieSupport=1#.VBMBfldXci.
Kenya National Bureau of Statistics (KNBS) and ICF Macro (2010). *Kenya Demographic and Health Survey 2008–09*. Calverton, Maryland: KNBS and ICF Macro.
Kenya Research Situation Analysis of Orphans and Vulnerable Children: Kenya Country Brief; Boston University, Center for Global Health and Development in collaboration with University of Nairobi, Institute for Development Studies, The (August 2009).
KNBS (2009). Kenya demographic and health survey 2008–2009. Kenya National Bureau of Statistics. http://dhsprogram.com/pubs/pdf/FR229/FR229.pdf.
Nyumbani (n.d.). http://www.nyumbani.org/.
Republic of Kenya Office of the Vice-President and Ministry of Home Affairs (2005). National Policy on Orphans and Vulnerable Children 2005.
Roby, J. and Shaw, S. (2008). Evaluation of a community-based orphan care program in Uganda. *Families in Society*, 89(1), 119–28.
SOS (2008). Child rights based situation analysis of children without parental care or at risk of losing parental care in Kenya.
UNAIDS (2011). The Kenya AIDS epidemic: Update 2011. Office of the President National AIDS Control Council. http://www.unaids.org/en/dataanalysis/knowyourresponse/countryprogressreports/2012cuntries/ce_KE_Narrative_Report.pdf.
UNAIDS (2012). http://www.unaids.org/en/dataanalysis/knowyourresponse/countryprogressreports/2012/countries/ce_KE_Narrative_Report.pdf.
UNCRC (2004). A summary on the rights under the Convention on the rights of the child. http://www.unicef.org/crc/files/Rights_overview.pdf.
UNDP (2011). Millennium development goals: Status report for Kenya. Ministry of State for Planning, National Development and Vision. http://www.ke.undp.org/content/dam/kenya/docs/MDGs%20Report/Kenya%20MDGs%0Status%20Report%202011.pdf.
UNDP (2012). Report on the Regional Dialogue on Women's Political leadership. Nairobi, Kenya: Author. http://www.ke.undp.org/content/dam/kenya/docs/Democratic%20Governance/UNDP%20championing%20womens%20leadership%20booklet3%20(1).pdf.

UNDP (2013). The rise of the south: Human progress in a diverse world. Human Development Report. http://hdr.undp.org/sites/default/files/Country-Profiles/KEN.pdf.

USAID (2013). Report to the people: The U.S.-Kenya partnership. http://www.usaid.gov/sites/default/files/documents/1860/USAID%20Kenya%202013%0Annual%20Report.pdf.

World Bank (2014). Kenya: Country at a glance. http://www.worldbank.org/en/country/kenya.

World Health Organization (WHO) (2012). Kenya: Health profile. http://www.who.int/gho/countries/ken.pdf?ua=1.

Chapter 4

The Living Arrangements of Vulnerable Children in Zambia

Margaret Lombe and Theresa Lungu

Introduction: Country Profile

Zambia is a landlocked country in south-central Africa. It covers 752,618 km^2. The country, formerly known as Northern Rhodesia, was a colony of the British government from 1886 until 1960 when it gained its independence. The country's official language is English. Zambia borders the Democratic Republic of the Congo to the north, Tanzania to the north-east, Malawi to the east, Mozambique, Zimbabwe, Botswana and Namibia to the south, and Angola to the west. The country's population stands at 13.8 million and is comprised of approximately 72 ethnic groups, most of which are Bantu-speaking. About 61 percent of the population are young people aged between 10 and 29 years. This sizable young population presents unique challenges in that future wellbeing is linked to the healthy development of people in this group.

Zambia is a democratic country with a multiparty political system. It has enjoyed relative political and economic stability since independence. Unlike many countries in sub-Saharan Africa, Zambia is highly urbanized with 44 percent of its population concentrated in a few urban areas such as the capital city (in the south) and in towns along the Copper-belt in the north-west. This information is noteworthy in that available data suggests that the prevalence of HIV/AIDS in Zambia varies significantly according to geographical location, with the cities recording higher rates.

Zambia is endowed with mineral resources including copper, cobalt, zinc, lead, coal, emeralds, gold, silver and uranium. In fact, at independence it was classified among the richest nations in sub-Saharan Africa. However, the country's economy declined considerably in the years following independence. With the privatization of the mining sector in the 1990s, Zambia experienced a boom in foreign investment, leading to economic growth. This growth was further augmented by the government's support of the agricultural sector. As of October 2011, Zambia was classified as a lower middle income country (World Bank, 2013). Despite this, social conditions for most people remain challenging. Poverty is widespread, life expectancy is among the lowest in the world and the mortality rate is one of the highest—largely due to the prevalence of chronic illnesses such as HIV and AIDS, malaria and tuberculosis. Indeed, the country's life expectancy on average stands at 52 years, 51 years for males and 54 for females; HIV prevalence exceeds 10 percent; public expenditure on health was estimated to be 4.8 percent of the GDP in 2012; infant mortality stood at 64.61 per 1,000 in 2012; furthermore, over 64.3 percent of the population lives on less than US$1.25 per day (World Bank, 2005). Further, it is important to note that as of 2007, 20 percent of households in the country were female-headed (MFNP, 2008). Eighty-two percent of the female-headed households are extremely poor as compared to the general population (UNICEF, 2008).

Definitions of Concepts

A number of definitions exist to delineate children experiencing adversity. A comprehensive appraisal of these is important and will help set the tone for this chapter. It is well understood that definitions often affect policy decisions and responses to a given phenomenon. Zambia has a dual legal system—permitting the application of customary and statutory law. Operationally, in Zambia, there are distinct active definitions of child, orphan and vulnerable child (Understanding Children's Work, 2012). For example, customary law defines a child anyone who has not yet attained the age of puberty—which is understood to be below the age of 14 years. The constitution of the Republic of Zambia provides multiple definitions, which are embodied in various articles. A child is defined as anyone under the age of 18 years (see Article 45). The Marriage Act, on the other hand, sets the age of 21 as the age of legal sexual consent.[1] The definition of child in Zambia is broad and loaded; it includes babies, toddlers, older children and adolescents. Indeed, the definition of child suggest that people categorized as children are entitled to certain protections as a result of their vulnerable status. It also implies that, by default, an individual above the age of 18 is an adult capable of taking care of herself despite the fact that the age of majority, legally, is set at 21 years (IRIN, 2011). The definitions offered also reveal the lack of a standard with respect to how to define a child in Zambia. Undeniably, the absence of clarity in definition is worthy of note; it may encourage misinterpretation of the law and may compromise its implementation, placing children at a disadvantage.

UNICEF and other major international organizations define an orphan as a child below the age 18 who has lost a parent/s. By this definition there are currently over 153 million orphans in sub-Saharan Africa, Asia, Latin America and the Caribbean (UNICEF, 2012). Within this group are children characterized as single orphan—indicating loss of one parent; and double orphans—indicating loss of both parents. This definition contrasts with concepts of orphan utilized

1 Whereas the penal code criminalizes any carnal knowledge of a girl under the age of 16 years, customary law allows marriage with the consent of parent or guardian for a girl of 14 years.

in countries of the global north, where a child must have lost both parents to be viewed as an orphan. It is important to note that, in most cases in sub-Saharan Africa, if a child has lost one parent to AIDS, the likelihood of the other parent to be HIV positive and eventually die of the disease is fairly high (Grassly et al., 2005). According to the Guidelines on Construction of Core Indicators established by UNAIDS (2010), the definitions of orphan encompasses children aged 10–14 years as of their last birthday who have lost both parents. The age range of 10–14 is used because younger orphans are more likely to have lost their parents recently, hence significant detrimental effects of the loss on their education would have had little time to materialize.

The observed difference in terminology needs to be underscored in that it often has implications for policies and programming for children experiencing vulnerability. For example, orphan statistics presented by UNICEF may be interpreted to mean that there are 153 million orphans worldwide who may be living alone and therefore in need of special care (UNICEF, 2012). This misunderstanding may lead to policy initiatives that focus on providing care for individual children. Similarly, responses may be instituted that focus on supporting families and communities in which orphans are nested, overlooking the child. To capture this reality, the compromise has been the introduction of the concept of OVC that encompasses vulnerability among children.

So then, who is a vulnerable child? In Zambia, a vulnerable child is categorized as a child below the age 18 who has a chronically ill (sick for three or more consecutive months within the last 12 months) parent or who lives in a household where an adult has been chronically ill or has died (Republic of Zambia, 2009). In addition to this, other factors that lead to vulnerability among children include poverty, hunger, lack of access to services, inadequate clothing and shelter, overcrowding in households and deficient caretakers (Skinner et al., 2006). Vulnerabilities that are specific to children include disability, physical or sexual violence and severe chronic illness.

In Zambia, children living in female-headed households or elderly-led households were found to be more food insecure as compared to other households (FAO, 2001). As a result children in these households are often malnourished. In Zambia, approximately 52 percent of under-five mortality has been due to malnutrition. As of 2008, 45 percent of children under five are stunted, 5 percent wasted and 19 percent underweight (UNICEF, 2008). In addition, poor quality of life makes this population of children susceptible to a myriad of diseases, such as pneumonia, diarrhea, acute respiratory infections and tuberculosis, all of which cause high rates of child mortality.

Specifically in the case of Zambia, many children are affected by the HIV/AIDS pandemic. These children are exposed to significant amounts of stress and trauma due to unmet social needs, death of parents, discrimination and added burden of work, which limits their overall capacity and wellbeing (Skinner et al., 2005; UNGASS, 2011; UNICEF, 2008).

Overview of the Issue

The first case of HIV/AIDS infection in the country was reported in 1984. Since then, infection rates have increased rapidly with the adult HIV prevalence rate peaking at about 16 percent, in the 1990s, and stabilizing at about 14 percent since then. As of 2013, 14.3 percent of Zambia's total population was infected with HIV. Available data suggests that the prevalence rates in Zambia vary significantly according to age, gender and geographic location. Levels of infection are notably higher among young people between the ages of 15 and 24. According to a Zambia country report, in the year 2008–9, approximately 30 percent of individuals in urban areas between ages 15–24 were HIV infected, compared to 16 percent in rural Zimbabwe (UNGASS, 2011). This holds true for children as well (UNGASS, 2011). This observation may imply that urban areas are likely to have more OVC than rural areas. About 4 percent of people living with HIV and AIDS are children aged 0–14 (AIDS, 2006; UNGASS, 2011).

HIV prevalence tends to be higher among young women. Globally, there are 7.3 million women between the ages of 15 and 24 living with HIV and AIDS, compared with 4.5 million men within the same age group. In sub-Saharan African countries, such as Ethiopia, Malawi, Tanzania, Zambia and Zimbabwe, young women between the ages of 15 and 19 are more likely to be infected, with an HIV prevalence of 5.7 percent compared to 4.7 percent among young men.

Existing data on the subject reveal that HIV and AIDS account for half of the estimated 1.3 million orphans and vulnerable children in Zambia. More specifically, this figure represents between 13 and 27 percent of all children below the age of 15 who have lost either one or both parents (CSO, 2009; UNICEF, 2003; Government of the Republic of Zambia, 1999). Further, about 19 percent of OVC in the country may be classified as double orphans. Double orphans are particularly vulnerable compared to children who have at least one parent living (Republic of Zambia, 2009).

Data from UNICEF indicate that half of the OVC in sub-Saharan Africa are fairly young, falling under the age of 10. More specifically, about 30 percent are aged between 6 and 10 while 18 percent are under the age of 5 (UNICEF, 2003), with the mean age estimated to be 6.2 years (Mugabe et al., 2002). In the case of Zambia, while a fair amount of data exists on OVC, there is a dearth of data that accurately reflect the demographic characteristics of this group. This makes correct presentation of a comprehensive picture challenging. According to statistics provided by UNICEF, on average only 2 percent of children are orphaned before their first birthday, where as 25 percent are orphaned between the age of 0–4 years, 35 percent between age 5–9 years and 50 percent are orphaned between 10–14 years of age as a result of the HIV/AIDS epidemic (UNICEF, 2003). Furthermore, compared to children in rural localities, urban children are more likely to be orphaned or vulnerable (16 percent vs. 27 percent). Another factor of note in Zambia is the bias in delivery of services for OVC, which seems to favor urban areas because the majority of public, private and civil society organizations are located in these areas (Republic of Zambia, 2010).

Issues/Problems Experienced by OVC in Zambia

Challenges faced by children classified as OVC are many. To adequately capture these, we organize them under four broad categories: health, psychosocial, economic and social welfare.

Health

Orphaned and vulnerable children generally face several constraints with regards to healthcare in Zambia. Prominent among these are inadequate healthcare, gaps in the supply of drugs, lack of information on the availability of services, and misinformation about HIV/AIDS and treatment options. Several national and international initiatives have been put into place to tackle the issue of HIV/AIDS. The National AIDS Surveillance Committee along with the National AIDS Prevention and Control Program has been in existence since 1986. The government recently developed National HIV/AIDS Strategic Frameworks for 2001–3, 2002–5 and 2006–10. These strategies have helped to set up support structures, which aim at planning and coordinating multi-sectoral responses to the epidemic. The most recent 2006–10 framework focused on intensifying prevention, expanding treatment, mitigating socio-economic impact, decentralizing and mainstreaming efforts, improving monitoring and integrating advocacy and coordination of various sectors (USAID, 2009). Since 2009, there has been significant progress in the number of adults who are able to access antiretroviral treatment (ART) as well as the adoption of World Health Organization (WHO) guidelines and availability of treatment for prisoners. These initiatives have an overall objective of expanding access to appropriate care, support and treatment for people living with HIV and AIDS, as well as TB, STIs and other opportunistic infections (UNGASS, 2011). In addition, international organizations such as PEPFAR, Global Fund, World Bank, UNAIDS, and other agencies have been providing monitory as well as skill based support to deal with the issue of HIV/AIDS in Zambia. However, effort targeting infected and affected children remains minimal country-wide (UNICEF, 2008). Indeed, existing evidence points to the fact that OVC have inferior access to healthcare compared to other children. They are less likely to initiate and complete the immunization protocol for their age, they are less likely to receive medical attention for common infectious and non-communicable diseases, and they are likely to experience delayed development or malnutrition (Center for Global Health and Development, 2012).

In recent years, the Zambian government has put in place policies eliminating user fees for healthcare services for children, allowing universal access to healthcare for children (Government of Zambia, 2006–10). This has been lauded as a successful policy across the country. However, the National Action Plan for Children in Zambia, which was launched towards the end of 2007, reported that access to essential healthcare services by children still remains low (Cheelo et al., 2010). The observed trends may be especially true for OVC who lack adult care. Many children in this category do not have the means to access public health facilities, which may be located at a great distance from the child's residence. Further, it may be that parents or guardians of OVC may be unable (too ill) to take them for medical care. Further, in many instances, the supply of services provided is often outpaced by the growing population of OVC.

Moreover, whereas availability of health services may be widespread in localities with more health facilities, rural areas still lag behind as they generally have fewer facilities, which are often poorly managed and/or equipped. Furthermore, the few health centers that exist in rural areas are not easily accessible because they are still far from where most rural dwellers reside. Indeed, people in rural areas have to travel long distances to get to the health centers. This picture suggests that the healthcare needs of OVCs may not be adequately met by the existing policies and infrastructure.

Psychosocial and Emotional Needs

It is common knowledge that OVCs experience unimaginable trauma through witnessing the suffering and eventual loss of a parent/s. The emotional burden of caring for a terminally ill parent/s may be unbearable, taking away stability and leaving affected children with unanswered questions about their future and own mortality. Further, not only do children who live in heavily affected areas contend with the death of their parents, they may also face the death of younger siblings as well as friends and close relatives. Despite this, the psychosocial impact of HIV/AIDS and its correlates on children are often overlooked. Indeed, while a number of programs addressing the material needs of orphans and vulnerable children have been put in place, there is little emphasis on helping children cope with the trauma associated with witnessing the deaths of family members. Furthermore, the psychological impact of HIV/AIDS on the young is often misunderstood. This is particularly the case in the school environment where frequent tardiness may be punished without an investigation of factors that may have triggered the behavior. Similarly, affected children may be censured for poor academic performance with no exploration of whether or not this is linked to trauma resulting from the children's challenging experiences.

In the past few years, attention has begun to focus on training teachers to identify grief-related behaviors. Statements from teachers who have completed grief-identification training suggest that their training has been useful and has enabled teachers to understand behavior previously conceptualized as deviant or problematic (Nzioka and Ramos, 2008). Programs are also being developed that enable children to play, a luxury for many orphaned and vulnerable children. It is well known that children affected by HIV/AIDS often begin to assume adult responsibilities, such as earning wages, caring for the terminally ill, and cultivating the land at an early age; leaving them with little to no time for recreational activities.

Psychosocial support is also overlooked with respect to caregivers. Reports of elderly grandmothers caring for numerous children with little to no income are not uncommon. These caregivers are often exhausted and overworked. It's important to note that in many parts of Zambia, especially in rural areas, the elderly have no social security or retirement benefits. As a result, children under their care are likely to be vulnerable, uneducated and malnourished. Recently, community-based organizations have begun to organize in support of caregivers. An example of this is a model in which elderly caregivers are provided additional support to improve their ability to cope with their caregiving roles. In addition, they are also given respite time, through participation in relaxation exercises, and engaging in leisurely community activities (Reddy et al., 2009). Support groups are also beginning to form to discuss and find solutions to other psychosocial problems experienced by the caregivers of OVC.

Economic

Despite reclassification of Zambia as lower middle income country (see World Bank, 2011), the majority of Zambians are considerably poor (Zambia Demographic Health Survey, 2007). Available data suggests that most households are not able to adequately meet their basic needs. The situation is often drastic for children who are orphaned and forced to live in single-parent homes, households headed by a child and for children living on the street. Indeed, incidents of poverty are known to increase dramatically upon the loss of a parent/s. Factors associated with the noted decline include loss of income resulting from diversion of resources to meet healthcare expenses, weak attachment to the labor market (in a monetary driven economy this is key for participation) and property grabbing.

Poverty among OVC is associated with heightened levels of food insecurity—resulting in chronic malnutrition. According to Global Action for Children (2010), malnutrition is one of the elevated risks experienced by orphaned and vulnerable children in Zambia. Evidence suggests that about 32.6 percent of OVC in Zambia are likely to go without food for a whole day because there is no food in the house. As a result of inaccessibility to food, many children suffer from malnutrition, stunting and wasting.

Poverty among OVC has also been linked to poor access to healthcare services. As noted, children in this group are less likely to initiate and complete the immunization protocol for their age, they are less likely to receive medical attention for common infectious and non-communicable diseases, they are likely to experience delayed development or malnutrition (Center for Global Health and Development, 2012). Despite waiving health-related fees, OVC are unable to access health services due to myriad causes including lack of knowledge, transportation, supervision or general support and awareness.

In addition, poverty has pushed a significant proportion of vulnerable children into the labor market to help supplement household resources. In fact evidence indicates that about 54 percent of OVC have worked for money—with boys reporting a higher likelihood of having worked previously compared to girls (Ngunga et al., 2014). Most of these children are to be found in the informal/alternative labor force characterized by unregulated and unsafe working conditions.

In the past few years, the Zambian government has committed itself to the alleviation of suffering among children. Steps taken by the Zambian government include the National Child Policy, a draft for a National Plan of Action for OVC, minimum standards of care, and the establishment of a district level coordinating mechanism (USAID, 2009). Measures have also been put in place to help curb food insecurity and nutrition problems in the country (UNGASS, 2011). Income transfers and educational vouchers have been introduced to help vulnerable children. Additionally, policies eliminating user fees for healthcare services for children have been established, allowing universal access to healthcare for children (Government of Zambia, 2006–10). Despite this, challenges still exist. The problem of the feminization of poverty and its spillover effects on children has become critical. In a recent study conducted by the Center for Global Health and Development (2012), it was found that poor OVC households are twice as likely to be female-headed households as compared to non-OVC non-poor households. Access to essential healthcare services by children, especially those in rural areas, child-headed and female-headed households, continues to be low (UNICEF, 2008).

Social Welfare

The country has a welfare strategy (the HIV Policy) for the care of orphans and other vulnerable children. The main objective of the HIV Policy is to strengthen the care and support structures for OVC through community-based interventions. Two ministries, including the Ministry of Sports, Youth and Child Development (MSYCD) and the Ministry of Community Development and Social Services (MCDSS) have the task of providing support for OVC in Zambia. More specifically, the MSYCD controls legal issues pertaining to protection of rights of children while the MCDSS addresses the delivery of basic social services. The National HIV and AIDS Strategic Framework are also responsible for the protection and provision of support for orphans and vulnerable children. In addition, Zambia has developed the Child Policy, an additional instrument addressing OVC issues. Moreover, a five-year national strategic plan on OVC and district level coordinating mechanisms for OVCs is currently underway in some districts (IMF, 2007). Further, at the national level, a Parliamentary Caucus on Children has also been established. In 2009 the Parliamentary Caucus Working Group began developing work plans, sourcing funding for a coordinator, and designing a pilot project to integrate issues of children into constituency development plans. At the district level, District AIDS

Task Forces (DATFs) and District Welfare Assistance Committees (DWACs) have been implemented to address challenges faced by OVC.

Notwithstanding the aforementioned, the most significant government response to the OVC crisis has come from the MCDSS, through the Public Welfare Assistance Scheme established countrywide. Their main goal has been to provide social protection to OVC by meeting their basic needs such as education, healthcare and good nutrition. To ensure equity in the delivery of services, the MCDSS has developed guidelines pertaining to management of the welfare assistance schemes, evaluation of vulnerability, and documentation of beneficiaries as well as assessment of the impact the support is having at individual, community and national levels. Plans to implement a comprehensive cash transfer scheme providing vulnerable families with a monthly income supplement to help lift them out of extreme poverty are in progress across the country. Another initiative, at the community level, is the National AIDS Strategic Framework (NASF), which focuses on:

1. protection and provision of support to orphans and vulnerable children;
2. provision of social protection for people made vulnerable by HIV/AIDS; and
3. promotion of food security and income/livelihood generation programs for OVC and their caregivers.

Through these schemes, a significant number of OVC (about 29 percent) have been reached with external support and care (NAC, 2009). However, challenges in the area of care of orphans and vulnerable children remain. The OVC situation appears to be developing into a deepening crisis as funding and programming is failing to keep pace with the magnitude of orphans who need care and support (UNAIDS et al., 2004). Female-headed households, characterized by limited resources, continue to be the primary caregivers for OVC. Further, NGOs are still the primary actors in the area of mitigating HIV-related needs of orphans and other vulnerable children in Zambia. Moreover, the issue of sustainability for community-based programs continues to be a challenge. There is also a marked bias favoring urban areas in the provision of services for OVC. This is mainly because the majority of civil society organizations are located in urban areas. Another setback has to do with the weak monitoring and evaluation systems aimed at capturing data on the welfare of OVC. Indeed, reliable data on the numbers of OVC is not readily available.

Overall, a significant number of children classified as vulnerable continue to experience stigma, abuse and exploitation. They are also known to have inadequate shelter and work to meet their basic needs, such as food and clothing. Further, their access to clean safe water or basic personal hygiene is not guaranteed (see Figure 4.1 for an overview of problems experienced by OVC).

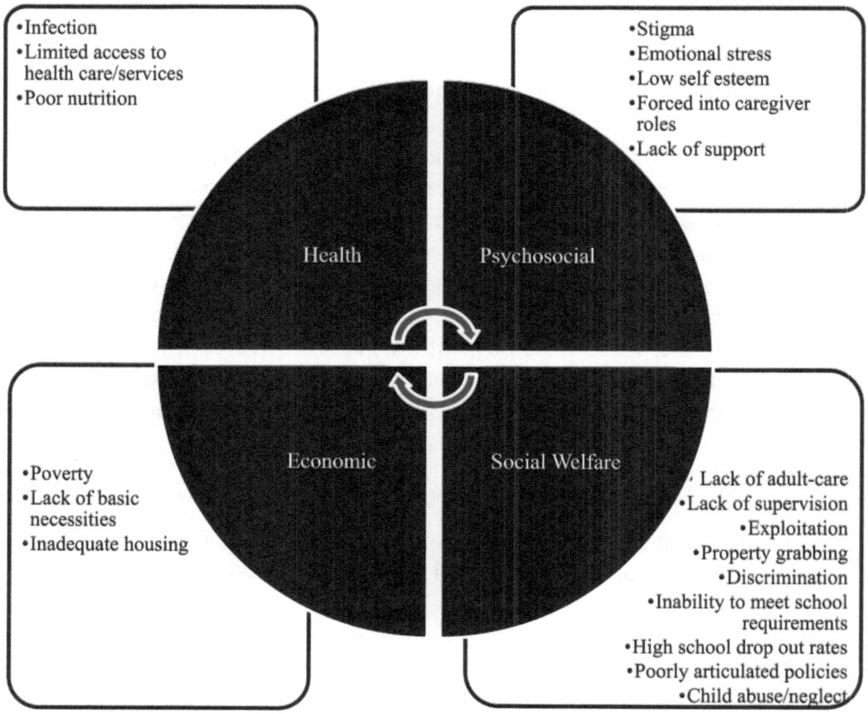

Figure 4.1 Problems experienced by OVC in Zambia
Source: Author.

Education

The Zambian government has taken action to address educational challenges with respect to OVC. This effort has been channeled, for the most part, through the Ministries of Education and Sport along with Youth and Child Development. One aspect of this has been the introduction of free education for vulnerable children in primary schools and a bursary scheme to increase access to secondary schools. Along with the noted interventions, the Ministry of Education has put in place policies that mandate the teaching of sex education in schools. Schools are required to include life skills related to HIV and AIDS education in their curriculum. The policy, however, does not cover the distribution of condoms to school-going children despite research evidence suggesting that school-going children are likely to be sexually active and engage in risky sexual encounters (Siziya et al., 2008; UNGASS, 2011). Another policy undertaking has been the implementation of a comprehensive national child policy through the MSYCD. The primary goal of the policy has been to provide guidelines on OVC support with regards to schooling.

Evidence suggests that the coverage of these initiatives has been minimal. This observation is problematic in that education is associated with numerous social benefits for both the individual and society. The importance of education for OVC is well documented (Argall and Allemano, 2009; Badcock-Walters, 2008; Bhargava, 2005; Boler and Carroll, 2005; Evans and Miguel, 2007; UNDP, 2013; UNGASS, 2011). School attendance is said to be one of the strongest remedies to a child's sense of loss, insecurity and anxiety. School is characterized by well-established routines—features likely to give a child experiencing instability and trauma a sense of normalcy. School serves as a social milieu in which the orphaned child can relate to peers and adults in a protected environment. School has potential to help the child develop a renewed sense of efficacy in relation to life, restoring confidence and sense of purpose. It may also be the one place where children get accurate information on HIV/AIDS. Moreover, school, for vulnerable children, may serve as a safe haven protecting them from abuse, hazardous labor and sexual exploitation (Lombe and Ochumbo, 2008). Furthermore, as has been observed by various social commentators, education may be the only means through which a vulnerable child can lift himself or herself out of poverty. Most importantly, education is a human right to which every child is entitled. It is also an essential precondition for the attainment of civil and political liberties (Human Rights Watch, 2005).

Legal and Policy Frameworks for OVC Care

Zambia's legal tradition is composed of a dual system consisting of traditional/customary law and statutory law. This is evident in various spheres including policies and legal framework put in place to safeguard the welfare of children. At the present time, Zambia does not have a comprehensive act to uphold the welfare of children. However, efforts to draft a statute, which comprehensively addresses the needs of children, are underway (Sloth-Nielsen, 2008). Through the MCDSS, the Zambian government has put in place measures for the protection of the welfare of children. Primary among these are the following:

- Affiliation and the Maintenance of Children Act;
- Adoption Act;
- Family Environment and Alternative Care Act;
- Juveniles Act;
- Employment of Young Persons and Children Act.

The main objectives of these instruments are to underscore rights pertaining to children, to set out guidelines for the care and protection of children, to define parental/adult responsibilities and rights, and to prevent child abduction and maltreatment. In general, the legal framework puts emphasis on four key principles. These consist of: (1) the best interests of the child; (2) non-discrimination; (3) the right to life, survival and development; and (4) respect for the views of the child. Below we review legal guidelines that relate to the care of children with a specific focus on orphaned and vulnerable children.

Articles 32–36 of the Juvenile Act of 1964 (amended in 1994). This Act is designed to safeguard the interest of children placed in institutional care. It articulates circumstances under which a child can be placed in institutional care. These include abandonment, and neglect or abuse, death of parents or guardians and juvenile delinquency. The Act also provides guidelines on who can/cannot foster a child in Zambia. Specifically, persons from whose care a child/children have previously removed are deemed to be unstable/unfit to care for a child, any person who has been convicted of an offence, persons living in premises declared as unsuitable—e.g., over-crowded, unsanitary, dangerous, and persons with situations defined as detrimental to the best interest of the child, e.g., age of caregiver, caregiver health, misconduct of caregiver, such as negligence, immorality, criminal conduct or any reason that define him/her as unfit to care for a child/children.

The Act also establishes guidelines with respect to creation of homes/orphanages for children. Among the requirements is presentation of a month's notice prior to establishment of the home. Procedures for periodic review of cases involving children placed in institutional care also exist. These serve to highlight the general circumstances of the child, foster parents and the community with the view of reintegrating the child into mainstream society. Further, institutions so established are subject to periodic inspection by a Juvenile Inspector.

Article 20 of the Family Environment and Alternative Care Act emphasizes parental responsibilities and the importance of family environment in the upbringing of children. It also underscores the state's obligation to provide special protection to children deprived of a family environment—e.g., through placement either with the extended family or foster care and provision of grants.

In general, the people of Zambia see the family as the basic social unit for the care, protection and nurturing of children. Indeed, the principle of investing in the welfare of children is very strong across the country. For example, under customary law, parents are obliged to provide for their children. This is also strongly emphasized by traditional norms and values. Among the Bemba-speaking people of northern Zambia there is a saying linking this investment to the future wellbeing of the caregiver "*Mayo mpapa naine kakupapa*"—meaning "Care for me now, I will care for you in your old age." This idea is common across ethnic groups in Zambia.

In recent years the problem of poverty and HIV/AIDS has made it especially challenging for provision of this Act to be satisfactorily realized. Indeed, the capacity of parents to provide adequately for their children has been severely compromised. Governmental assistance, for the most part, has been inadequate.

Adoption Act—54 (1964/5 Amended in 1994)

One of the primary mandates of the Department of Social Welfare in the MCDSS is to create permanent family units for children through adoption. It has to be noted that the country has no policy or legal provision to guide the adoption of vulnerable children specifically. The provision currently in place offers guidelines with respect to who can adopt a child in Zambia and defines the conditions under which this can occur. The Act underscores the following:

1. attainment of the age of 21 if the person initiating the adoption is related to the child;
2. age limit—the adoptee/s be at least 21 years older than the child to be adopted;
3. gender requirement—that the adoptee be of the same gender as the child—in case of sole adoptees;
4. infant to be in continuous care and possession of adoptee for at least three consecutive months before the adoption order;
5. giving three months' notice of adoption to the Commissioner prior to adoption proceeding;
6. parental consent to be given where parents are alive (legal guardian); and
7. protection of the best interest of the child at all times.

Living Arrangements of OVC in Zambia

As observed, much of the burden of caring for OVC falls heavily on the extended familial systems of care and communities, accounting for about 90 percent of OVC care (UNICEF, 2003). Fostering through the extended family, in Zambia, represents an informal temporary arrangement outside of state regulation, which is often crisis-driven and may be the only form of care available to OVC. For the most part, women and the elderly (e.g., aged grandparents) are more likely to take responsibility for fostering and provision of psychosocial support to OVC. This is especially the case for double orphans. Another common avenue utilized for the care of OVC is the single-parent household often headed by a maternal caregiver. OVC are also to be found in publicly regulated institutions such as orphanages and children's villages. Child-headed households, a new phenomenon in the country, have also emerged as a type of sociological domiciliary composed of children often from the same family unit (Meintjes et al., 2010). Another type of living arrangement for OVC is the street—depicting a situation in which children experiencing homelessness reside on the streets (including unoccupied dwellings and wasteland) of big cities. An overview of the different living arrangements of OVC in Zambia is presented next.

Fostering in Zambia

Guidelines around fostering either through traditional kinships of care—extended family—and statutory or state-regulated foster institutions are loosely defined. With respect to fostering through state-regulated institutions, care is structured in accordance with the provisions of chapter 53 of the Juveniles Act (The Zambian Law Database, 2008). The Department of Community Development and Social Services supervises and monitors the placement and situation of children in alternative care. Before alternative care is even considered for a child, social inquiries are made concerning the child's cultural, social and religious background. It is important to note that the Juvenile Act requires that this be taken into account and that children be placed in settings that are close to their normal living environment. In fact, when separation is necessary, custodial care by a member of the extended family is the preferable option. Institutionalization of children, even in temporary shelters, is often the last resort.

In terms of customary law, the nuclear and extended familial systems are the two main family structures available to a child in Zambia. Largely because of settlement patterns dictated by employment, the nuclear family tends to be more pronounced in urban areas while the extended family is prominent in rural areas. Customary law respects the responsibilities, rights and duties of parents, the extended family and community to rear their children. The State party also acknowledges that nurturing and socialization of a child lies in the exclusive domain of the family with elders in the community taking moral authority over this. Indeed, it is generally accepted, especially in rural localities, that the elders in society possess knowledge and information about culture, child development and the evolving capacities of the child, and therefore are better positioned to transmit knowledge and values. The rearing of a child, in many parts of Zambia, is a communal responsibility, hence the adage "It takes a village to raise a child." In fact, this obligation is deeply rooted in the tradition, culture and family values of Zambians.

Customary law acknowledges and respects the customs and child-rearing practices of all ethnic groups in the country. In the case of the death of a parent, custody of the children is generally granted to the remaining parent (UNICEF, 2003). In instances where both parents have died, custody may be given to a close relative—an aunt/uncle or grandparents. The authority to grant custody of orphaned children rests with the kinship—at times only with close family members. The kinship, generally, deliberates on the suitability of the guardian before custody is awarded. Attention is given to factors such as financial capability and moral standing. To our knowledge, neither customary nor statutory law offers guidelines with respect to fostering of children by the extended family. Indeed, there are no legal guidelines to determine who can/cannot be given custody of orphaned children despite the fact that the majority of orphaned children remain in the care of the extended family. Although data on children fostered through the extended family are not readily available because of the fluidity of the practice and the lack of documentation, current estimates indicate that about 30 percent of fostered children are raised by an aunt, uncle, grandparent or other close relative.

For years, the extended family has provided a traditional safety net, and has sheltered children from suffering the full impact of social, economic or physical deprivation, particularly when biological parents are absent and adult care unavailable. In the majority of cases, orphans who are fostered through the extended family are treated with fairness and dignity (Roby, 2011). Anecdotal evidence, on the other hand, suggests that in situations where caregivers are overburdened and family resources constrained, fostered children may experience unjust treatment (Subbarao et al., 2001). Evidence points to the fact that orphaned children are more likely than non-orphans to be stunted, to be out of school, and to carry heavier loads of physical work (Center for Global Health and Development, 2012; FHI and SCOPE OVC, 2002). Evidence also suggests that fostered children generally perceive themselves as being treated unjustly. They may be the last in line when food is being distributed (or, even worse, they may be denied food), the last to have their school requirements met, and may even experience maltreatment, e.g., required to perform the bulk of household chores and are severely punished for minor wrongdoings (FHI and SCOPE OVC, 2002).

Moreover, evidence points to the potential for children so affected to experience adjustment problems. This has been linked to the fact that decisions about placement of orphans with a relative are seldom taken with consultation of the children involved. Further, the decision may require separating siblings and relocating them to new physical locations, homes and schools. Indeed, orphaned children, in general, are rarely incorporated into a foster family as a unit due to limited capacity (Government of Zambia, 1999). Research evidence also suggests that HIV/AIDS has weakened the capacity of the extended family system, resulting in acute vulnerabilities for orphaned children (UNICEF, 1999). Furthermore, in Zambia, like in many parts of sub-Saharan Africa, it is often poor families with limited resources who assume the additional responsibility of caring for orphaned children. This is further compounded by the lack of a social safety net.

The Grandparent-Headed Household

An overview of the living arrangement of vulnerable children in grandparent-headed households, a common living arrangement for OVC, is used to illustrate the traditional kinship of care. In Zambia fostering by the extended family accounts for about 33 percent of the living arrangements of OVC (Mugabe et al., 2002). Such households generally form when a family has experienced the death of two or more adult caregivers, compelling grandparents to step-in to care for orphaned children. Many of the elderly caregivers lack the physical and health resources, energy and vigor to adequately care for a second, and sometimes even a third, family late in their lives. Coupled with this is the lack of income to meet basic necessities. Indeed, primary caregivers in this group are not gainfully employed, often have no access to retirement benefits and do not have access to public safety nets. They may also be dealing with the emotional trauma of the loss of their own security through the death of their own child/children. The issue of their own care, in a country that does not have a comprehensive welfare system, may arise—who would provide for their upkeep in their old age? The orphans for whom they care are likely to face the possibility of experiencing loss yet again when the elderly caregiver dies. For these reasons, the welfare of children in grandparent-headed households may be highly compromised. Notwithstanding these challenges, fostering by grandparents is one of the most stable forms of caregiving available to OVC in the country. It ensures orphaned children stay in one housing unit, experience adult supervision and emotional wellbeing.

Children in Orphanages and Other Supported Facilities

As observed, the prevalence of HIV and AIDS coupled with relentless poverty has severely compromised the traditional systems of care, forcing a significant proportion of children to slip through the cracks. Some of these have found their way into orphanages. Although orphanages for the most part adequately cater for the child's material needs, they are not an appropriate first-line response to the OVC crisis in sub-Saharan Africa in general and Zambia in particular. For one thing, institutional care tends to cost much more compared to a corresponding level of care within a family or community (Larson, 2010; World Bank, 2001). Further, the absorptive capacity of such institutions is so low that they can only take in a small fraction of the children. It is also generally understood that orphanages are not a culturally appropriate response to the OVC crisis. Indeed, they fail to adequately address the child's emotional and psychosocial (developmental and long-term) needs. In addition, there is the question of whether or not orphanages reflect lack of will by government and other responsible institutions to act on behalf of vulnerable children. Moreover, as has been argued by social commentators, the beneficiaries of this enterprise are rarely the vulnerable children purported to be served (Barnett and Whiteside, 2002). It is well known that the overhead of running an orphanage is much higher than the dollar/kwacha value that accrues to each child. Moreover, orphanages are rarely located in villages where they may be more needed. The sentiments expressed here are not, in any way, intended to diminish the support orphanages have provided to vulnerable children in Zambia. To the contrary, this is an attempt at underscoring the fact that regulated care is but a partial response to the problem.

In response to the challenges alluded to in this discussion and the enormity of the needs of OVC, an alternative quasi-institutional model has emerged in Zambia. This is largely made up of community-based day centers where children can receive respite and care including meals, education and medical attention while they continue to live in their own homes. Where need be, adult supervision is provided to ensure that the living conditions of children living alone are reasonable. In fact, there is some subjective evidence to indicate that some communities, by consensus, have appointed designated caregivers to monitor and support children who live on their own. A good example of this approach, in Zambia, is the Kenneth Kaunda Children of Africa Foundation, which has established day-care centers in five high-density locations of Lusaka to provide care to younger children between the ages of three and nine. People from the community, for the most part, assume the responsibility of the day-to-day running of the day centers. This model looks promising. However, it is fairly recent; hence, it lacks sound empirical grounding.

Other Living Arrangements: Single-Parent Households, Child-Headed Households and Children on the Streets

Single-parent households

With respect to OVC, single-parent households are usually formed upon the death of a parent and are dependent on whether or not the surviving parent resolves to maintain the household for herself/himself and offspring/s. Although a male may head such households, female-headed households are the most common (UNICEF, 2003). In many parts of Zambia, when the mother dies, children are likely to be dispersed among relatives to ensure they are well cared for. This is normally the case when surviving children are very young. Another common occurrence following the death of a mother is that the father remarries. Hence, households with children headed by a male without a female partner or spouse are uncommon.

Data on the prevalence of female-headed households are hard to come by. Our estimate, however, indicates that this is a fairly common living arrangement for OVC in Zambia and accounts for roughly 22 percent of OVC living arrangements (UNGASS, 2011). Female-headed households are often characterized as vulnerable mainly because women tend to be disempowered and seldom have access to land and other productive resources. Their livelihood usually depends on small-scale horticultural and agricultural ventures, low-paid domestic jobs, petty trading and other activities in the secondary labor market. There is also some evidence suggesting that mothers and female offspring in such households might turn to prostitution and petty thieving to supplement their income and household resources (Runhare and Gordon, 2004; UNICEF, 2003). Children in female-headed households are generally characterized as vulnerable in that such households tend to be fragile economically. This, however, might be one side of the story. The other side might be that such households offer orphaned children a solid social bond guaranteeing stability, security and love.

Child-headed households

As is the case in parts of sub-Saharan Africa, communities in Zambia are finding creative ways to cope with the OVC crisis. One of these has been the emergence of a relatively new social structure known as the child-headed household. Current estimates are that child-headed households consist of about 2 percent of all household types nationwide (Meintjes et al., 2010). These households are composed of sibling units who have who have lost adult members—mother and father. Child-headed households may also have an adult who may be too infirm to take on adult roles and to contribute to the household's livelihood. The structure of authority, in child-headed households, is organized primarily around the oldest child, often by unspoken consensus. This child, often under the age of 18, may assume economic and quasi-parenting responsibility for the younger siblings.

The phenomenon has come about mainly as a response to the loss of parents and the escalating levels of vulnerability/poverty that make it difficult for familial networks to absorb orphaned and vulnerable children. The fact that siblings have lived and worked together in caring for their sick and/or dying parents serves as an empowering and unifying mechanism. Further, in the process of care, the oldest child may have experienced adultification—referring to the process through which a child is socialized to take on adult roles (see Nebbitt and Lombe, 2010). This arrangement enables children to stay together and avoid disruption of the family unit. It also ensures, to some extent, that the children do not suffer maltreatment at the hands of relatives. Notwithstanding the above, child-headed households are likely to experience extreme poverty and other vulnerabilities. Indeed, the risks faced by OVC children in such households are heightened, as they are forced to navigate life without adult care and supervision. Whilst data on the impact of HIV and AIDS on children is available, disaggregated information on OVC by living arrangement is not readily available. Most of the data at hand is subjective, collected for other purposes such as monitoring the impact of public assistance schemes on OVC. The observed data limitation on the subject presents a challenge in presentation of a comprehensive overview of the phenomenon of children in child-headed households in Zambia.

As suggested by the name, children in child-headed households live under the care of a sibling—typically another child. In general, children heading such households are fairly young, with the youngest being between the ages of 10 to 12 years (Foster et al., 1997). They often have weak or no connection to the kinship of care. Indeed, the primary caregiver—a child—is often ill equipped to provide guidance, support and protection to younger siblings. In fact, there is some evidence to suggest a correlation between lack of parental supervision and compromised welfare. For example, Schönteich (2000), points to poor/low parental supervision and involvement as one of the key predictors of delinquency and violence in later life. Lack of parental supervision is connected to poor educational attainment and health outcome (Dawson, 1991; Foster and Williamson, 2000; Fan and Chen, 2001; Theilman et al., 2012). This and similar observations fuel concerns that the lack of adult care in OVC households has the potential not only to negatively impact the welfare of children in such households but may lead to an increase in crime and delinquency in the long-run.

Moreover, there is also concern that leaving children under the care of "another child" who is unprepared to play the role of parent may translate into poorly socialized young people, threatening the social fabric and the stability of society. Indeed, social commentators suggest that the absence of adult supervision that characterize children in child-headed households has the potential to rob them of role models, nurturing and the opportunity to acquire cultural values which are essential for social participation (Foster et al., 1997; Thurman et al., 2006). Similar observations have also been made by the United Nations Food and Agricultural Organization (FAO) which has noted that HIV/AIDS, in rural localities, has disrupted mechanisms for transferring knowledge, values and beliefs from one generation to the next, compromising the transfer of farming skills (FAO, 2001).

In addition, there is the issue of lack of capacity to navigate challenges of providing for household with regards to financial, material and social resources. Child-headed households are often characterized by poverty due to lack of attachment to the labor market and any source of income generation. Evidence on the subject suggests that, due to lack of resources, children in such households have developed mechanisms to cope with vulnerability. These may consist of reducing the number of meals per day as well as the quantity of food intake. Another area that may be affected is health related spending as well spending associated with school requirements. To make ends meet, they may be forced to sell off household goods and productive assets. They may even resort to prostitution and begging from relatives, friends and/or neighbors.

Furthermore, on top of the emotional toil of losing their primary caregivers, children in child-headed households suffer from numerous adverse social consequences. They are likely to be malnourished and under-fed (Foster and Williamson, 2000); report higher proportions of child labor (Mugabe et al., 2002); are likely to experience stigmatization and discrimination and may also arouse sentiments of fear and suspicion in others. Child-headed household are also at risk for emotional and sexual abuse and exploitation (UNICEF, 1999), as well as greater risk for HIV infection due to their vulnerability. Access to school, for the most part, is precarious for children in child-headed households. The responsibilities of caring for younger siblings may force the caregiver to give up school (Ainsworth and Filmer, 2002). Furthermore, the household may not have enough resources to meet school-related expenses. It could also be that everyone in the household has to work to help generate the resources needed for survival. In fact evidence exists to support the observations made here (ILO, 2003; UNICEF, 2003).

In general, the experience of children in child-headed households is characterized by vulnerability. They are likely to face food insecurity, poor health, poor education outcomes as well as lack of psychosocial support. They also have a lower likelihood to develop into independent, well- adjusted adults with the capacity to be successful and contribute to the general welfare of their country. Their situation is further compromised by the lack of governmental programs/ initiatives that specifically target their predicaments. In rural communities, such households survive through active community care/support. Indeed, networks of caring adults have come together to provide guidance as well as material and emotional support. In the context of the city, assistance may be provided through drop-in centers like the Children Village alluded to earlier.

Children on the streets

This is a term used to define children experiencing homelessness who primarily reside on the streets (including unoccupied dwellings and wasteland) of big cities. They often experience inadequate protection and supervision. Their primary source of livelihood is the street (De Benitez, 2007; Ray et al., 2011; Barker and Knaul, 1991). Street children differ in age, gender, ethnicity and social class. In general, they are fairly young, with the majority in the age group of 11–18 years. Boys make up a significant number of children who live on the streets (Beasley, 1999). Existing evidence suggests that although girls live on the streets as well, their numbers tend to be smaller. A possible explanation for this is that girls tend to be more "useful" in the home, taking care of younger siblings and helping with household chores. Nevertheless, girls have a greater vulnerability to trafficking for commercial sexual exploitation and/or other forms of child labor.

Children who are vulnerable to street life include those who have been abandoned by their families or sent into cities because of a family's acute poverty, often with hopes that a child will be able to earn money for the family and send it home. Children who run away from home or children's institutions frequently end up on the street since they rarely return home. In several parts of Africa, disabled children may be abandoned, hence are likely to be part of this group. In addition, refugee children and children in areas experiencing protracted conflict may be found in this group. Also likely to be part of this group are orphaned children.

The hidden and isolated nature of the phenomenon of street children makes accurate data difficult to gather. However, UNICEF estimates there are approximately 100 million street children worldwide with that number constantly on the increase. For example, there are up to 40 million street children in Latin America, and at least 18 million in India (UNICEF, 2006). In the case of Zambia, the number of street children is estimated to be between 35,000 and 75,000 (Zambian Ministry of Sport, Youth and Child Development, 2004). This represents an increase of about 0.9 percent in the 1990s to 1.6 percent in 2004. Many children in this group come from poor families and families affected by HIV, poverty and other shocks. Although a significant number of children in this category live on the street, most of them are not orphans (Project Concern International Zambia and Lemba, M., 2002; UNICEF, 2006). In fact, USAID has divided street children into four main categories, which are commonly used worldwide. These consist of:

- Children of the streets; describing children whose primary residence is the street.
- Children on the street; referring to children who have families but regularly return every night to the street because of poverty, overcrowding, sexual or physical abuse at home.
- Children in families that live on the street: describing children who live on sidewalks or city squares with the rest of their families.
- Children in institutionalized care: identifying children from a situation of homelessness who are at risk of returning to a life on the street.

Existing evidence suggests that street children often operate in groups, united by their common need for survival (UNICEF, 2005). Street children are vulnerable and have unstable lifestyles. Indeed, their survival is mainly through alternative activities such as street work, begging, petty theft and prostitution for girls. They are also unlikely to be in school, further compromising their life chances. Their limited/lack of healthcare services and inadequate living conditions is linked to increased susceptibility to chronic illnesses such as respiratory infections, gastrointestinal disorders, and sexually transmitted diseases, including HIV/AIDS. Further, children fending for themselves are likely to experience severe food insecurity and may be engaged in exploitative child labor. Children in this group may experience heightened mental health problems resulting in part from insecurity and their nomadic lifestyle. Public perception of these children is often negative—they are seen as a public nuisance and a risk to the safety of the general public. Although vulnerable, children in this group are unlikely to receive governmental support—they may be afraid to seek help or may not be aware of it.

Homelessness and street life have extremely detrimental effects on children. For the most part, in Zambia, the general response to the plight of children on the street is to protect the public by removing them. Effort has, in recent years, focused on limiting their crime involvement through provision of basic necessities and rehabilitating them into mainstream society (Wernham, 2004). Key players in this effort have been government ministries such as the MSYCD, non-governmental and faith-based organizations as well as other civil society institutions.

Challenges to OVC Care

In this section we summarize a few of the many challenges to OVC care. For years, the extended family has provided a traditional safety net, and has sheltered children from suffering the full impact of social, economic or physical deprivation, particularly when biological parents are absent and adult care unavailable. In the majority of cases, orphans who are fostered through the extended family are treated with fairness and dignity (Roby, 2011). Anecdotal evidence, on the other hand, suggests that in situations where caregivers are overburdened and family resources constrained, fostered children may experience unjust treatment (Subbarao et al., 2001). Research has found that orphaned children are more likely than non-orphans to be stunted, to be out of school, and to carry heavier loads of physical work (Center for Global Health and Development, 2012; FHI and SCOPE OVC, 2002). Research has also revealed that fostered children generally perceive themselves as being treated unjustly. They see themselves as being the last in line when food is being distributed (or, even worse, they may be denied food), last to have their school requirements met, and the person likely to experience maltreatment, e.g., required to perform the bulk of household chores and be severely punished for minor wrongdoings (FHI and SCOPE OVC, 2002). Moreover, evidence points to the potential for orphaned children to experience adjustment problems. This may be linked to the fact that decisions about placement of orphans with a relative are seldom taken with consultation of the children involved. Further, the decision may require taking apart siblings and relocating them to new physical locations; homes and schools. Indeed, orphaned children, in general, are rarely incorporated into a foster family as a unit due to limited capacity (Government of Zambia, 1999). The extended family system continues to weaken, resulting in acute vulnerabilities for orphaned children (UNICEF, 1999). Furthermore, in Zambia, like in many parts of sub-Saharan Africa, it is often poor families with limited resources who assume the additional responsibility of caring for orphaned children. This is further compounded by the lack of a social safety net. Attention could be devoted to provision of support to families caring for OVC.

Another challenge in OVC care involves the lack of data aggregated by gender, age and vulnerability status. This makes it difficult to effectively monitor and understand the nature, extent and magnitude of problems faced by vulnerable children in Zambia. It also compromises responses to the plight of OVC. Coupled with this is the absence of coordination among the different actors in the ecosystem serving vulnerable children—making it difficult to avoid replication and resource wastage. This is especially troubling given the limited resources and the magnitude of the problem. A comprehensive system to track resource use and beneficiaries of these organizations may be needed to curb this. Another aspect of this is the need for improved surveillance systems, enhancing knowledge creation with respect to what is known about the scale, scope and impact of alternative care for OVC. Indeed, the gaps in knowledge severely undermine the ability to understand the magnitude of the OVC crisis and responses to care needs and effectiveness of current care initiatives.

Over the past few years the Zambian government, non-governmental organizations, and other civil society agencies have increased their attention to the plight of OVC, especially homeless and street children. However, as the number of this disenfranchised population continues to grow dramatically, effort often lags behind need. Furthermore, monitoring of facilities caring for vulnerable children, although mandated under the Juvenile Act, at most is inadequate or nonexistent, jeopardizing the welfare of children in foster care.

At the policy level, lack of clearly articulated guidelines for OVC care continues to be a challenge. Coupled with this are the problems inherent in the duality of the country's legal system—customary and statutory law. Indeed even basic elements, such as the definition of a child, is open for debate because of discrepancies in customary and statutory law. Also, the absence of legal guidelines to control the fostering of children by the extended family remains a challenge. While traditionally, the familial system had a built-in mechanism of control/sanction, this is no longer available for most children experiencing vulnerability, especially in urban locations. In traditional Zambian society, the welfare of fostered children was ensured through mechanisms of accountability such as proximity to each other—the extended family lived in the same village, which provided strong moral values as well as strong ties to the family. A comprehensive children's policy to safeguard the welfare of children characterized as vulnerable is needed to ensure children are adequately protected. This might require dialogue between the two systems—customary and statutory. Indeed, definitions of concepts like child and vulnerability may need to be standardized across the country to allow for effective responses to the plight of vulnerable children. Political will to implement and revise existing policies so they reflect the reality of the OVC situation is needed.

Conclusion

In the past few decades vulnerability among children in Zambia has increased considerably. The government and non-governmental organizations have put together a number of responses to alleviate suffering among children. These initiatives have helped improve the lives of vulnerable children and have enhanced community willingness to take care of OVC. Indeed, formal support has led to a reduction in psychosocial stress in households, particularly ones headed by elderly women (Horizons, 2005; UNAIDS, 2005). However, across the board, only 19.1 percent of rural and 11.6 percent of urban OVC report receiving assistance from sources outside of the household and kinship network (UNAIDS, 2005). Moreover, as far as children in child-headed households are concerned, vulnerability continues to be a problem. The same can be said about children on the street. Currently, the number of children residing on the street and in child-headed households is small. Evidence, however, suggests that this number is likely to grow as the capacity of the extended family to absorb orphaned children continues to diminish. Furthermore, leaving the responsibility to care for children to other children may have significant implications for the welfare of children and society as a whole. Rectifying the situation will require an accurate evaluation of the phenomenon of vulnerable children in Zambia. The observed data limitation on the subject presents a challenge in this regard and points to the need for continued monitoring of the situation of children made vulnerable by HIV and AIDS. Alongside this is the need for proactive policies and legal frameworks that accurately reflect the experiences of vulnerable children.

Bibliography

Ainsworth, M. and Filmer, D. (2002). Poverty, AIDS and Children's Schooling: A Targeting Dilemma. Evidence from 28 Developing Countries. PowerPoint presentation, World Bank, Washington, January 8, 2002.

Argall, J. and Allemano, E. (2009). *Case Study. Schools as Centres of Care and Support. Responding to the Needs of Orphans and Other Vulnerable Children in Rural Areas*. Tunis Belvedere: ADEA.

Badcock-Walters P. (2008). *Supporting the Educational Needs of HIV-Positive Learners: Lessons from Namibia and Tanzania*. Kloof: EduSector AIDS Response Trust.

Barker, G. and Knaul, F. (1991). *Exploited Entrepreneurs: Street and Working Children in Developing Countries*. New York: Childhope USA.

Barnett, T. and Whiteside, A. (2002). *AIDS in the Twenty-First Century*. Basingstoke: Palgrave Macmillan.

Beasley, R. (1999). On the Streets. *Amnesty Magazine*, April 1999. http://www.amnesty.org.uk/news/mag/.

Bhargava, A. (2005). AIDS epidemic and psychological well-being and school participation of Ethiopian orphans. *Psychology Health and Medicine*, 10(3), 263–75.

Boler, T. and Carroll, K. (2003). *Addressing the Educational Needs of Orphans and Vulnerable Children*. London: Action Aid International and Save the Children UK.

Brody, A.B. (2002). Combating HIV/AIDS: Intervention Strategies, Impact Mitigation and Policy Issues. Paper presented to International Conference on "Commitment to Combat HIV/AIDS," University of Swaziland, Kwaluseni Campus.

Center for Global Health and Development (2012). Impact on Health Status of Orphans and Vulnerable Children (OVC) in Namibia of Mobile Primary Care Clinics Provided by the Mister Sister Public Private Partnership. Washington, DC: USAID Project SEARCH.

Center for Global Health and Development (2012). The Wellbeing of Orphans and Vulnerable Children and Their Households in Four Districts of Mozambique. Research Report, Boston University-OVC CARE Project. USAID.

Cheelo, C., Chama, C., Pollen, G., et al. (2010). Do user fee revenues matter? Assessing the influences of the removal of user fees on health financial resources in Zambia. Working Paper No. 2010/1. Lusaka, Zambia: University of Zambia, Department of Economics.

CSO (2009). *Zambia Demographic and Health Survey 2007*. Calverton, MD: ORC-Macro, with Central Statistics Office, Lusaka.

Dawson, D.A. (1991). Family Structure and Children's Well-Being: Data from the 1988 National Health Interview Survey on Child Health. *Journal of Marriage and Family*, 53(3), 573–84.

De Benitez, S.T. (2007). *State of the World's Street Children: Violence*. London, UK: Consortium for Street Children.

Donovan, P. (2000). The Impact of HIV and AIDS on the Rights of the Child to Education; Discrimination and HIV/AIDS-related Stigma and Access to Education—the Response. Paper presented at SADC-EU Seminar on the Rights of the Child in a World with HIV and AIDS. Harare, Zimbabwe, October 23, 2000.

ECA (Economic Commission for Africa) (2001). *The African Development Forum 2000: Leadership to Overcome HIV/AIDS*. Addis Ababa: Economic Commission for Africa.

Evans, D.K. and Miguel, E. (2007). Orphans and Schooling in Africa: A Longitudinal Analysis. *Demography*, 44(1), 35–57.

Fan, X. and Chen, M. (2001). Parental Involvement and Students' Academic Achievement: A Meta-Analysis. *Educational Psychology Review*, 13(1), 1–22.

FAO (2001). *The Impact of HIV/AIDS on Food Security*. Committee on Food Security, 27th Session, Rome, May 28–June 1, 2001. Rome: FAO.

FHI (Family Health International) and SVOPE OVC (2002). Psycho-social Baseline Survey (data highlights). FHI, Lusaka, March 2002.

Foster, G. and Williamson, J. (2000). A Review of Current Literature of the Impact of HIV/AIDS on Children in Sub-Saharan Africa. *AIDS*, 14(suppl. 3), S275–S284.

Foster, G., Makufa, C., Drew, R., and Kravlovec, E. (1997). Factors Leading to the Establishment of Child-Headed Households: The Case of Zimbabwe. *Health Transition Review*, 2(7), 155–68.

Global Action for Children (2010). Orphan and Vulnerable Children. http://www.globalactionforchildren.org.

Government of the Republic of Zambia (1999). *Orphans and Vulnerable Children: A Situation Analysis, Zambia 1999*. Joint USAID/UNICEF/SIDA Study Fund Project.

Government of Zambia (1999). *Zambia: A Situation Analysis of Orphans*. Joint USAID/UNICEF/SIDA Study Fund Project. Lusaka: UNICEF.

Government of Zambia (2006–10). National Health Strategic Plan (NHSP).

Grassly, N.C. and Timmaeus, I.M. (2005). Methods to estimate the number of orphans as a result of AIDS and other causes in Sub-Saharan Africa. *Journal of Acquired Immune Deficiency Syndromes*, 39(3), 365–75.

Horizons (2005). Exploring the role of family caregivers & home-based care programs in meeting the needs of people living with HIV. http://www.popcouncil.org/uploads/pdfs/horizons/hbccrgvrsa.pdf.

Human Rights Watch (2005). Letting Them Fail: Government Neglect and the Right to Education for Children Affected by AIDS. *Human Rights Watch*, 17(13A), 1–59.

Hunter, S. and Williamson, J. (1997). *Developing Strategies and Policies for Support of HIV/AIDS Infected and Affected Children*. Report to USAID.

ILO (2002). *HIV/AIDS and Child Labour in Zambia: A Rapid Assessment*. Geneva-Lusaka: International Programme on the Elimination of Child Labour, ILO.

ILO (2003). *Investing in Every Child: An Economic Study of the Costs and Benefits of Eliminating Child Labour*. Geneva, Switzerland: Author.

IMF (2007). IMF Country Report No. 07/276 Zambia: Poverty Reduction Strategy Paper. Washington, DC: Author.

IRIN (2011). Zimbabwe: Cash transfers target vulnerable children. http://newirin.irinnews.org/.

Kaleeba, N., Kadowe, J.N., Kaliaki, D., and Williams, G. (2000). *Open Secret: People Facing up to HIV and AIDS in Uganda*. Strategies for Hope Series, No. 15. London: ACTIONAID.

Larson, B. (2010). *A costing Analysis of a Household Economic Strengthening (HES) Program for Households Caring for Orphans and Vulnerable Children (OVC): A Case Study of Christian Aid's Community-based Care for OVC (CBCO) Program*. Washington, DC: USAID Project Search.

Lombe, M. and Ochumbo, A. (2008). Sub-Saharan Africa's orphan crisis: Challenges and opportunities. *International Social Work*, 51(5), 682–98.

Meintjes, H., Hall, K., Marera, D.H., and Boulle, A. (2010). Orphans of the AIDS Epidemic? The Extent, Nature and Circumstances of Child-Headed Households in South Africa. *AIDS Care: Psychological and Socio-Medical Aspects of AIDS/HIV*, 22(1), 40–49.

MFNP (2008). Economic Report 2007. Lusaka: Ministry of Finance and National Planning. In Component Report for the Situation Analysis of Children and Women in Zambia (2008), *Household Income and Poverty*. Lusaka: RuralNet Associates Limited.

Ministry of Health (2007). Assessment of the Health Information System in Zambia. http://www.nmcc.org.zm/files/ZambiaHISAssessmentReport.pdf.

Mugabe, M., Stirling, M., and Whiteside, A. (2002). Future Imperfect: Protecting Children on the Brink. Discussion paper presented to Africa Leadership Consultation: Acting for Children on the Brink. Johannesburg.

NAC (2009). NARF summary report 2008.

Nebbitt, V. and Lombe, M. (2010). Urban African American Adolescents and Adultification. *Families in Society: The Journal of Contemporary Social Services*, 91(3), 234–40.

Ngunga, M., Chapman, J., Chariyeva, Z., and Kamwanga, (2014). *A Situation Analysis of STEPS OVC Program Beneficiaries: Analyses of Endline Data*. Lusaka, Zambia: USAID/STEPS OVC.

Nzioka, C. and Ramos, L. (2008). *Training Teachers in an HIV and AIDS Context: Experiences from Ethiopia, Kenya, Uganda and Zambia*. Paris: International Institute for Educational Planning.

Project Concern International Zambia and Lemba, M. (2002). Rapid Assessment of Street Children in Lusaka. New York: UNICEF. http://www.unicef.org/evaldatabase/files/ZAM_01-009.pdf.

Ray, P., Davey, C., and Nolan, P. (2011). *Still on the Street: Still Short of Rights*. Plan and Consortium for Street Children.

Reddy, S.K., Parsons, H.A., Elsayem, A., et al. (2009). Characteristics and correlates of dyspnea in patients with advanced cancer. *Journal of Palliative Medicine*, 21(1), 29–36.

Republic of Zambia (2009). Zambia Demographic and Health Survey 2007. Lusaka, Zambia: Author. http://www.dhsprogram.com/pubs/pdf/FR211/FR211 [revised-05-12-2009].pdf.

Roby, J.L. (2011). *Children in Informal Care Alternative Care*. UNICEF: Child Protection Section.

Runhare, T. and Gordon, R. (2004). *The Comprehensive Review of Gender Issues in the Education Sector*. UNICEF/MoESC. http://www.unicef.org/evaldatabase/files/Gender_Review_REPORT_final.pdf.pdf.

Schönteich, M. (2000). Age and AIDS: A Lethal Mix for South Africa's Crime Rate. Konrad Adenauer Stiftung Occasional Papers, Johannesburg, June 2000.

Siziya, S., Muula, A.S., Kazembe, L.N., and Rudatsikira, E. (2008). Harmful Lifestyles' Clustering among Sexually Active In-School Adolescents in Zambia. *BMC Pediatrics*, 8(6).

Skinner, D., Mfecane, S., Gumede, T., et al. (2005). Barriers to accessing PMTCT services in a rural area of South Africa. *African Journal for AIDS Research*, 4(2), 115–23.

Skinner, D., Tsheko, N., Mtero-Munyati, S., et al. (2006). Towards a definition of orphaned and vulnerable children. *AIDS Behavior*, 10(6), 619–26.

Sloth-Nielsen, J. (2008). A Developing Dialogue—Child Rights, Children's Law and Economics: Surveying Experiences from Southern and Eastern African Law Reform Processes. *Electronic Journal of Comparative Law*, 12(3).

Subbarao, K., Mattimore, A., and Plangemann, K. (2001). *Social Protection of Africa's Orphans and Other Vulnerable Children. Issues and Good Practices. Program Options*. Africa Region Human Development Working Paper Series, Africa Region, The World Bank. Washington, DC: The World Bank.

Theilman, N., Ostermann, J., Whetten, K., et al. (2012). Correlates of Poor Health among Orphans and Abandoned Children in Less Wealthy Countries: The Importance of Caregiver Health. *PLoS ONE*, 7(6), e38109, doi:10.1371/journal.pone.0038109.

Thurman, T.R., Snider, L., Boris, N., et al. (2006). Psychological Support and Marginalization of Youth-Headed Households in Rwanda. *AIDS Care: Psychological and Sociological Medical Aspects of AIDS/HIV*, 18(3), 220–29.

UNAIDS (2005). *HIV/AIDS, Gender and the Care Economy: The Social and Economic Impact of HIV/AIDS*. Geneva, Switzerland: UNAIDS Inter Agency Task Team on Gender and HIV/AIDS.

UNAIDS (2010). Indicator Standards: Operational Guidelines for Selecting Indicators for the HIV Response. Geneva, Switzerland: Author. http://data.unaids.org/publications/irc-pub06/jc935-3onesinaction_en.pdf.

UNAIDS, UNICEF and USAID (2002). Children on the Brink 2002: A Joint Report on Orphan Estimates and Program Strategies. Washington, DC: TvT Associates. www.usaid.gov and http://www.unicef.org/media/publications/children_on_brink.pdf.

UNAIDS, UNICEF and WHO (2002). *Young People and HIV/AIDS: Opportunity in Crisis*. Geneva: UNAIDS; New York: UNICEF; Geneva: WHO.

UNAIDS, USAID and UNICEF (2004). *Children on the Brink 2004: A joint report of new orphan estimates and a framework for action*. New York: UNICEF. www.unaids.org.

Understanding Children's Work (2012). *Towards Ending Child Labour in Zambia: An Assessment Of Resource Requirements*. Rome, Italy: Author.

UNDP (2013). *Millennium Development Goals: Progress Report—Zambia*. Zambia: UNDP.

UNGASS (2001). *Declaration of Commitment on HIV/AIDS*. United Nations General Assembly, 26th Special Session, June 27, 2001. New York: United Nations.

UNGASS (2011). *Zambia Country Progress Report: Monitoring the Declaration of Commitment on HIV and AIDS and the Universal Access*. Submitted to the United Nations General Assembly Special Session on HIV and AIDS.

UNICEF (1999). *Children Orphaned by AIDS: Front-Line Responses from Eastern and Southern Africa*. New York: UNICEF.

UNICEF (2001). *Growing Up Alone: Childhood Under Siege*. London: UNICEF 2001.

UNICEF (2003). *Africa's Orphaned Generations*. New York: UNICEF.

UNICEF (2005). *Children Out of Sight, Out of Mind, Out of Reach*. New York: Author.

UNICEF (2006). *The State of the World's Children 2006: Excluded and Invisible*. New York: Author.

UNICEF (2008). *The State of the World's Children 2009*. New York: UNICEF.

UNICEF (2008). *Zambia: Situational Analysis of Children and Women 2008*. Zambia: UNICEF.

UNICEF (2012). *The State of the World's Children 2011 Adolescence: An Age of Opportunity*. NY, New York: Author.

USAID (2009). Research situation analysis: Zambia country brief. OVC-CARE Project, Boston University Center for Global Health and Development. http://www.bu.edu/cghd/files/2009/12/Zambia-Research-Situation-Analysis-Country-Brief.pdf.

USAID (2011). Zambia: Country development cooperation strategy 2011–2015. Washington, DC: Author.

Wernham, M. (2004). *An Outside Chance: Street Children and Juvenile Justice—an International Perspective*. London, United Kingdom: Consortium for Street Children.

World Bank (2001). *Costs of Scaling HIV Program Activities to a National Level in Sub-Saharan Africa: Methods and Estimates*. AIDS Campaign Team for Africa (ACTafrica), March 31, 2001. Washington, DC: The World Bank.

World Bank (2005a). *The OVC Tool Kit*. Washington, DC: World Bank.

World Bank (2005b). *The World Bank's Global HIV/AIDS Program of Action*. Washington, DC: World Bank.

World Bank (2011). Reproductive Health Glance Zambia. http://siteresources.worldbank.org/INTPRH/Resources/376374-1282255445143/Zambia52311web.pdf.

World Bank (2013). World Bank List of Economics. http://librarians.acm.org/sites/default/files/wdi2013.pdf.

Zambian Law Database, The (2008). Chapter 53 (Volume 5): The Juveniles Act. http://zamlaws.zambia.co.zm/laws_view.php?chapter=53.

Zambian Ministry of Sport, Youth and Child Development (2004). *Orphans and vulnerable children in Zambia*. Lusaka, Zambia: Author.

PART III
Responding to Orphaned and Vulnerable Children: An Overview of Public and Private Initiatives

Families and communities have been at the heart of responses to the needs of orphans and vulnerable children in sub-Saharan Africa. For the most part, these social entities have been left to tackle the problem with little formal support. In recent years, government ministries and schemes together with community-based, faith-based, and other civil society agencies have stepped up to address the challenge presented by OVC. Their efforts, although laudable, have been, to a large extent, inadequate and at times uncoordinated. In this section, we review these, their historical underpinning, challenges and implications for the welfare of OVC. The section is organized into three chapters. Each chapter examines the responses of key actors in a given setting, i.e. Botswana, Kenya, and Zambia. We also examine the extent to which children have participated in decision-making. A systematic review of the literature along with an appraisal of relevant government databases provides material for the three chapters.

Specifically, Chapter 5 illustrates responses of the government of Botswana and civil society to the plight of OVC in the country. Laws, policies and their implementation guidelines are analyzed for their comprehensiveness, relevance, and whether or not they are stagnant or progressive in addressing the complex situation of OVC and their caregivers. The existence or lack of laws and policies that reflect the international conventions, charters, and declarations on the rights of the child that the Botswana government has ratified or signed is examined. Programs geared toward the promotion of OVC's welfare, health and development as well as their impact are discussed. Chapter 6, on Kenya, gives an overview of responses to OVCs, the legal framework guiding these responses, and their historical evolution. The chapter also addresses challenges inherent in these policies and their implications. Data from the survey will be used to complement literature review. Chapter 7 presents a general picture of the situation of OVC in Zambia with respect to governmental and civil society's responses to their plight. An historic evolution of legislation implemented to safeguard the interest of OVC is given as background. International conventions and treaties the Zambian government has ratified with regards to children are examined. Public and private initiatives put in place to promote the welfare of OVC are discussed. The chapter also looks at the involvement of children, or lack of, in issues related to policy implementation and programming.

Chapter 5
Responses to Orphaned and Vulnerable Children (OVC) in Botswana

Naomi Seboni, Tapologo Maundeni, Ogar Rapinyana,
and Mosidi Tseleng Cynthia Mokotedi

Introduction and Background Information

Botswana, like many African countries, has experienced an increase in the numbers of OVC. The existence of children classified as vulnerable is not peculiar to contemporary Botswana society, it also prevailed in traditional societies. What is different is the official classification of children as vulnerable, the volume of children who need care, the circumstances leading to their vulnerability, and the resources available for their care. Like other African countries, Botswana is going through a process of rapid social, economic and cultural change. One of the characteristics of this change has been the disintegration of the extended family. Another has been reduction in the capacity of familial systems to cope with both the quality and quantity of care that OVC require (UNDP, 2000).

In traditional African societies,[1] for example, OVC were absorbed in the extended family system. Indeed, relatives were obliged to take care of people in need in accordance with the roles expected of each family member. Family members who were related to one another by blood, marriage or adoption lived together in the same compound or in the same part of the village. Their material and social needs (food, shelter, clothing and emotional support) were taken care of by the extended family as a whole (Schapera, 1984; Himonga, 1985). People complied with kinship obligations to a great extent because they feared and respected social sanctions. With the advent of colonialism, industrialization, migration, urbanization and the introduction of the money economy (rapid socio-cultural changes) the strong support system that prevailed in traditional societies no longer existed. As Himonga (1985, p. 256) observed:

> The above system of support and protection for women and children, being characteristic of a single traditional society, no longer exists under modern conditions.

---

1 Traditional Tswana society refers to Botswana prior to industrialization, urbanization and modernization. This was a society before the introduction of the money economy and the migration of people from rural to urban areas.

The same trend has also been noted by Ndulo (1984, p. 22) who rightly pointed out that:

> The joint family is in a state of decline and Africans are now enmeshed in an exchange economy. Development and industrialisation have caused an unreasonable breakdown in the traditional African social order. The society is now highly individualistic, competitive and acquisitive.

Another transformation resulting from this has been the disintegration of the system of residence; members of the same family group no longer live close together in the same household, ward or village. Some family members now work outside their villages or even outside the country and are not within the reach of senior family members who may want to enforce obligations of support (Molokomme, 1987). Furthermore, the high cost of living in towns and limited accommodation facilities may have restricted the extent to which people can help others.

In the context of contemporary Botswana, an orphan is defined as a child below the age of 18 years who has lost one parent (single orphan) or both parents (double orphan) (Government of Botswana, 2008a). A vulnerable child on the other hand is defined as any child under the age of 18 years who lives: in an abusive environment; in a poverty-stricken family and is unable to access basic services; or a child-headed household; with sick parents or outside family care; or who is HIV positive (Government of Botswana, 2008b). Part X of the Children's Act (2009) lists several groups of children as children in need of care. These include: children who have been abandoned, neglected, ill-treated or exploited and no suitable adult relative can be found who is willing and able to care for the child or his or her parents or other relatives have been found but are unwilling or unable to care for the child; as well as a child who has a disability and is subjected to discrimination or is deprived of proper parental care as a result of that disability. There is a dearth in reliable national figures that provide an accurate picture of the full population of abused, neglected and abandoned children in the country partly because each organization keeps its own figures, and they do not combine and share statistics. However, during the past few years, the Department of Social Services (DSS) has requested UNICEF to fund a national study on child abuse. It is hoped that this study will provide reliable data on the extent of child abuse in the country. Although there are no reliable figures on child abuse in the country, social workers and police officers as well as the scant available literature indicate that child maltreatment is increasing in the country (cf. Ministry of Local Government, 2001).

The purpose of this chapter is three-fold. First it provides an overview of challenges faced by OVC in Botswana. Second it analyses responses to OVC care and welfare. And lastly, it highlights recommendations with greater potential to improve/enhance the welfare of children classified as vulnerable. Issues covered in the chapter are guided by data gleaned from desk research. A review of documents (both published and unpublished) that focus on OVC in Botswana was done. Policy frameworks were also examined. Documents reviewed included key national legal and policy frameworks, reports on relevant international conventions as well as scholarly papers and information relating to OVC. In addition, national and international databases were accessed and reviewed for supportive data.

Country Background and the Magnitude of OVC

Brief background information about Botswana is crucial in order for readers to appreciate some of the issues discussed in this chapter. Since attainment of self-rule in 1966, the country has made strides in the provision of social, educational and health services. Life expectancy, health, mortality rates, literacy, nutrition and infrastructure have improved considerably (United Nations, 2004). The government has introduced free basic education (grades 1 through 7) for Botswana citizens. Further, school fees are highly subsidized at secondary school and children from poor families are exempted from paying school fees. The government also provides a primary healthcare system that offers essential health services in an evenly distributed and accessible way to all people. There is a clinic or health post within 5–8 km of every village, resulting in 89 percent of the population having access to healthcare (Shaibu, 2004). Children's access to primary healthcare services is boosted by the fact that healthcare services for children are free of charge.

Although Botswana has made progress in various respects and its rapid development has benefitted most of its population, the country has its own problems, mainly poverty, an increase in existing and emerging chronic illnesses such as HIV and AIDS, and communicable and non-communicable diseases (Republic of Botswana, 2004).

Botswana is one of the countries that have been hard hit by HIV and AIDS. Therefore, adults of child-bearing age continue to die in large numbers—leading to surges in numbers of orphans in the country. In 2001, for example, there were approximately 111,812 orphans in the country, representing about 15.2 percent of children below the age of 18 years (Central Statistics Office, 2003). In 2007, the number of orphans was estimated at 137,805, representing 17.2 percent of children below the age of 18 (Government of Botswana, 2008a). Current estimates are that about 44,000 children are orphaned (UNICEF, 2013). On a similar note, a total of 36,183 OVC were registered with the DSS (USAID, 2010a; UNICEF, 2011). These numbers are alarming and require urgent action from various stakeholders.

Challenges Faced by OVC

Orphans and vulnerable children face numerous challenges. In this section, only a few will be highlighted. It is well documented that one of the problems experienced by OVC is the loss of an important figure that the child is attached to. This pervades every aspect of the child's life: their emotional wellbeing, physical security, mental development, educational development and overall health. Children in this situation are also likely to be deprived of many of their basic human rights, e.g. rights to education, protection from harm, exploitation, discrimination, health and nutrition, (UNICEF, 2004). Such deprivation affects them in numerous ways.

A situational analysis of OVC in Botswana conducted in 2008 indicated that while the majority of OVC are happy in the homes they live in, concerns still exist. Many of these relate to treatment by caregivers, unfair allocation of resources (even when these belonged to the OVC), and lack of emotional support.

Orphans experience trauma and hardship as there is usually little family planning for the children's future (UNAIDS, 2004; USAID, 2004). It is often the case that when a parent or primary caregiver falls ill dependent children begin to take on a greater responsibility for income generation, food production and the care of younger family members. Consequently, their nutrition, healthcare, housing and clothing are compromised. Indeed, there is some evidence to suggest that OVC are also likely to: drop out of school; perform poorly in school; to be transferred to new schools after a guardian's death; experience property grabbing, abuse, stigma, isolation and emotional stress (Maundeni, 2006). Moreover, these children are likely to live in poverty (Government of Botswana/UNICEF, 2006). The observed trend is clearly illustrated in the words of a guidance and counseling teacher who taught in one of the schools surveyed by one of the authors:

> Children who are orphans do not live well. It is very painful to lose a parent when one is still young like these children. It affects them a lot, and this is exacerbated by the fact that orphans experience many problems both in school and outside. For example, some relatives do not treat orphans nicely, they discriminate against them. One day, one of the orphans just came to my office crying, she said other children were teasing her because she is an orphan, she revealed many other problems that she was going through as a result of her status as an orphan. I felt overwhelmed, I also felt that I did not have enough skills to counsel her … so I referred her to a social worker in the community.

The difficult circumstances confronting orphans affect them negatively. The negative effects take one or more of the following forms: depression, anxiety, unintended pregnancies, early marriages and deteriorating health conditions (*The Botswana Guardian*, December 1, 2000). In the long-term, these experiences negatively impact on the society at large. For example, children who experience dysfunctional childhoods are more likely to be unable to contribute meaningfully to national development when they reach adulthood, and may even create a dysfunctional environment for generations after them (Osei-Hwedie, 2000).

Lastly, one other challenge which commonly confronts OVC, but which is often overlooked by stakeholders, is frequent exposure to research interviews. In recent years, there has been an escalation of child-centered research in Botswana. By child-centered research, we mean research that involves children as respondents. Such research can focus on a wide range of issues. But this section is largely concerned with research focusing on children and psychosocial issues. While effort to generate knowledge should be encouraged, child-centered research may be problematic in that, as currently implemented, little attention is devoted to planning and preparing child-participants for such endeavors. In addition, monitoring guidelines to facilitate the conduct of ethical research are poorly defined (Maundeni and Levers, 2004). Available guidelines relate to research in general; the current structure assumes a focus on adults and does not specify any special protocol for research that focuses on the child as a subject in research.

Responses to the Challenges of OVC

Legal and Policy Frameworks that Guide Responses to OVC Care

Several pieces of legislation that aim to address the unique and multifaceted challenges faced by OVC prevail in Botswana. These include: The Children's Act of 2009; Children in Need of Care Regulations (2005); the Adoption Act (Cap 28:01); the Penal Code (CAP 08:01); as well as the Short-Term Plan of Action for OVC. These laws are reviewed below.

The Children's Act
This is the principal legislative governing the welfare of children. It is also seen as the main enforcement vehicle for the implementation of Botswana's obligations under the Convention on the Rights of the Child. The Act was passed in 2009. The Act aims to provide a protective environment for children. Following are its primary objectives:

1. Promote the wellbeing of children, families and communities in Botswana; provide for the protection and care of children where their parents have not made such provision, or are unable to provide that protection and care.
2. Protect children from harm, acknowledge the primary responsibility of parents and families to care and protect children, and support and assist them in carrying out that responsibility.
3. Acknowledge the role played by communities in promoting and safe-guarding the wellbeing of children and encourage and support them in carrying out that role.
4. Protect children from unlawful or exploitative labor practices (section 4).

The Children's Act also enshrines the best interest principle as being the paramount consideration in the care of children. This is in line with the requirements of the CRC and the ACRWC which underscore the best interests of the child as paramount. Section 5 of the Children's Act states that in assessing best interests the following factors are to be taken into consideration: the need to protect the child from harm; the capacity of the child's parents, relatives, or guardian or other person to care for and protect the child; the child's spiritual, physical, emotional and educational needs; the child's age, maturity, sex, background and language; the child's cultural, ethnic or religious identity; the likely effect on the child of any change in circumstances; the importance of stability and continuity in the child's living arrangements and the likely effect on the child of any change or disruption in those arrangements; any wishes or views expressed by the child given the child's maturity; any factor ensuring the wellbeing of the child. These factors are not exhaustive; any issues leading to the attainment of the best interests of the child should be taken into account.

Part X of the Children's Act contains numerous sections that focus on matters related to child protection. These include: definition of children in need of care; reporting of such cases; application of protection order; and the welfare of children with disabilities.

Overall, the contents of the Act are address key issues that are central to the protection of children. Moreover, they are aligned to the rights guaranteed under the CRC.

The Children in Need of Care Regulations (2005)

This legislation regulates foster care arrangements. Specifically it sets out guidelines for monitoring foster parents and families, screening parents of children in need of care, educating, and reviewing foster placements on a periodic basis (for details see World Fit for Children Mid-Term Review, 2007).

The Adoption Act: The third piece of law that addresses the needs of OVC is the Adoption Act (Cap 28:01). While this Act has good intentions, some of its contents are not relevant to the complex and multifaceted challenges faced by OVC because it is outdated since it was formulated in 1952—long before Botswana ratified the two major instruments on children's rights (i.e. the CRC and the ACRWC). It therefore needs to be reviewed to reflect the provisions of the above mentioned international treaties. Such a move will go a long way in ensuring that survival, development and participation rights are promoted, respected and fulfilled. In fact, proposals are underway to review the Adoption Act.

Policies

The Short-Term Plan of Action (STPA) is the major policy that addresses the needs of OVC in Botswana. The overall goal of the STPA is to "improve the socio-economic conditions of orphans by way of investing in human capital, within the broader context of sustainable human development" (Ministry of Local Government, 1999, p. 9). The specific objectives of the STPA are as follows:

1. Respond to the immediate needs of orphans.
2. Identify various stakeholders and define their roles and responsibilities in responding to the orphan crisis.

3. Identify mechanisms of supporting community-based responses to the orphan problem.
4. Develop a framework for guiding the long-term program development of orphans.

Under the STPA, orphans receive material assistance and psychosocial support until they reach the age of 18. Services stipulated under the STPA are largely provided by the government. However, several non-governmental organizations also offer services guaranteed under STPA.

Among the services provided for under STPA stipulation is provision of counselling to OVC. In reality, however, counselling is rarely offered mainly because of workload (social workers are overwhelmed with the volume of orphans) and skill limitations. Because of staff shortages that characterize human service agencies, a social worker may be responsible for covering multiple locations. For instance, in 2007, there were only 420 social workers employed by the local authorities in Botswana. The central government, NGOs, the private sector, hospitals and other government institutions only employ a small number of social workers. The few OVC who are fortunate enough to receive counselling are assisted on casework basis. Group work is rarely utilized due to factors such as rigid working hours for local authority social workers and the inability of people who are free after hours to come for group sessions.

In recent years, the Government of Botswana has put together financial assistance packages given to organizations servicing OVC. USAID (2010b) reported that "The total costs to Government for providing OVC services irrespective of service type is BWP 54 666 788 (US$ 7 822 817). The cost per child was BWP 11 624 (US$ 1,663) per annum" (p. 26) (see Table 5.1). It must be noted that food and nutrition accounted for 61 percent of total government assistance to OVC (USAID, 2010) (see tables 5.1 and 5.2).

Table 5.1 Summary of government total and unit costs

Type of cost	BWP	USD
Total costs	BWP 54,666,788	USD 7,822,817
Unit cost	BWP 11,624	USD 1,663

Source: Created using data from USAID (2010b, p. 114).

Table 5.2 Summary of government total costs by service area

Service area	Total costs (in BWP)	Total cost (in USD)	Percentage
Food and nutrition	BWP 33,307,535	USD 4,766,308	61%
Education	BWP 10,658,807	USD 1,525,275	20%
Shelter and care	BWP 7,292,320	USD 1,043,531	13%
Clothing and bedding	BWP 2,767,848	USD 396,079	5%
Psychological support (PSS)	BWP 640,278	USD 91,624	1%

Source: Created using data from USAID (2010b, p. 115).

In an effort to monitor the trends of OVC the government has employed desk officers at all districts to register children classified as vulnerable. This is seen as a crucial step in the planning process. Currently, according to the OVC Situation analysis report, about 92 percent of households receive food assistance for the care of OVC. Most of the recipients of food assistance are OVC registered through the orphan program. In addition vulnerable children are supported through the Destitute Policy which outlines assistance with food rations.

Response from NGOs and Other Civic Organizations

Several NGOs and CBOs provide various forms of assistance to OVC in the country. Examples of such organizations include: Stepping Stones International, Mahalapye Mothers Union, Childline-Botswana, SOS children's village, Silence Kills Support Group, Special Education Society, Tumelong Counseling Centre, Hajee Gulam Mustapha Chidren's Home, Kamogelo Day Care Centre and Mpule Kwelagobe Centre and Masiela Trust, among others. Programs and services provided include: integrating OVC in the school system; pre-school education; non-formal teaching for school dropouts and other out-of-school children; life skills training and educational support to OVC; fun days for all pre-school children in the community; income generation for support groups and youth groups; youth outreach and mobilization; feeding programs for day care; home-based care; support groups and counseling; psychological, spiritual help for OVC and their guardians; capacity building, networking, mentoring and teaching support, policy implementation (Government of Botswana, 2008a).

The civic organizations in Botswana work toward improvement of social and health outcomes of OVCs and they are well coordinated through an umbrella organization called Botswana Council of Non-Governmental Organizations (BOCONGO). Their interventions toward OVC draw upon the principles of CR's shadow report of 2004. Programing often takes into account the unique situation of OVC who have experienced emotional problems due to a double tragedy of losing a parent/parents and having HIV and AIDS infections. As Maundeni (2004) has observed, civic organizations have made significant headway in promoting awareness as well as providing support and care to vulnerable children.

These organizations play an important complementary role in responding to the plight of OVC; they supplement government effort. The existence of CBOs/NGOs/FBOs shows they are crucial government partners in providing services to OVC as they are able to reach the majority of children in need throughout the country due to their connection to the grassroots.

According to USAID (2010a; 2010b), NGOs provide a range of care and support services for OVC in Botswana. Table 5.3 shows the types of services offered by these organizations. The data have been disaggregated to show services provided by 15 district/local government agencies and 22 NGOs.

Table 5.3 Types of services provided to OVC by type of organization

Service provided	No. of organizations (N = 37)	No. of districts/local government agencies	No. of NGOs (N = 22)
Institutional care	4	1	3
Temporary housing/foster care	8	5	3
Obtains birth certificates/assist caregivers/parent obtaining birth certificates	12	7	5
Day care/nursery	14	2	12
Vocational training/income-generating activities	16	6	10
Access to legal protection	19	9	10
Register orphans/assist caregivers/assisting parents to register orphans	20	9	11
Provision of food basket	22	10	11
Health related services	24	9	15
Youth clubs	25	7	18
Material support/personal care	26	15	11
Education support	27	12	15
Psychosocial support/counseling	30	12	18

Source: Created using data from USAID Health Policy Initiative (2010a, p. 19 (p. 116)).

Kinship Care

Kinship care is another response that tends to benefit OVC in Botswana. In fact it is the one that is commonly used to cater for the needs of such children. According to the Department of Social Services (2005), at least 95 percent of orphans are absorbed within the kinship structures based on descent and marriage. Like in many African countries, kinship care is not regulated by formal institutions or by laws. Therefore, human service professionals such as social workers rarely intervene in the placement of children in kinship care because of the authoritative roles that relatives play in such placements. In varying degrees kin provide shelter, emotional support, educational support, spiritual support as well as moral support.

Traditionally, kinship systems emphasized sibling bonds, provided a sense of belonging, and gave support and security to members by sharing the little they had. When children are placed with people they know, Testa and Rolock (1999) argue that this is likely to reduce the possibility of depression and isolation that are consequences of separation, and offers growth and development within the context of a child's culture and community. Placement within the extended family is seen as important in that it strengthens the children's sense of identity and self-esteem which emanate from knowing their familial and communal culture (Testa and Rolock, 1999). Another advantage of extended family fostering is that it is culturally acceptable and assumed to be sustainable throughout a child's development, partially because communities will band together to support these households (Deininger et al., 2003). In most cases, children have found stability, love, and emotional support in relatives' homes (Maundeni and Malinga-Musamba, 2013).

Despite the positive role that kin play in the lives of children classified as vulnerable, for some children, kin have been sources of stress. For example, kin rarely consult children about where they prefer to stay following the death of their parent/s. Such decisions are largely handled by adult relatives (Maundeni and Malinga-Musamba, 2013). This practice partly arises from a community's lack of awareness of children's rights; as well as the culture of Botswana which tends to put emphasis on the saying that "children should be seen but not heard" (see Maundeni, 2002, for a detailed discussion of this practice). The exclusion of orphans in decisions about their living arrangements following the death of their parent/s is not fair and stands in violation of article 12 of the CRC, which states that "children not only have the right to articulate their opinions with regard to issues that affect them, but they also have a right to have these opinions heard." Another related and rather disturbing trend about kinship care is that, more often than not, relatives have a tendency to separate orphans (Maphalala, 2007). This step is taken mainly for economic reasons. Relatives contend that the high cost of living does not enable them to care for a large number of children, particularly when they have their own biological children to care for (Raditedu, 2004; Maphalala, 2007).

Another point to note in relation to kinship care is that, to a large extent, relatives are not trained or provided with the support to enable them to care for OVC adequately. This is not surprising taking into account the point made elsewhere in this chapter—that kinship care is not regulated by formal structures. Hence, a person with poor parenting skills may end up as primary caregiver to OVC. The absence of training for kin is one of the issues that need serious attention (Maundeni and Malinga-Musamba, 2013). This is particularly so because there is evidence indicating that kin are not able to address the emotional issues confronting orphans. For example, traditionally, in African society, people are not comfortable in disclosing information that is related to illness and death. Elders, including caregivers, provide a shield from what they assert to be the cruel facts of life, believing that this is in the child's best interest (Jacques, 2003).

Statutory Fostering

Statutory fostering represents transfer of parental roles to an institution. In Botswana, as of 2008, formal alternative caregiving arrangements for children in need of care included residential care as well as formal adoption and guardianship sanctioned by the courts. Formal adoption and guardianship are not common in the country (Maundeni, 2009a). In this section we provide an overview of institutional care.

Residential care facilities for children in need of care in Botswana are a relatively recent phenomenon. The first facility was established in 1987, and currently, there are about five such institutions in existence. Examples of these include Save Our Souls (SOS) villages,[2] the facility run by Childline Botswana, which was established in 2003,[3] as well as the Mpule Kwelagobe facility,[4] which started operating in 2000. Generally, these institutions are staffed by social workers. For example, the SOS villages—in different parts of the country—have employed a total of six social workers. Three of the six are directors while the other three provide direct psychosocial support services to residential children in need of care. Only one of these is institutions is fully funded by the government, the rest are funded by international and local NGOs (Maundeni, 2009a).

The institutional settings ensure that sibling units are kept together under the guidance of a house mother. In other words, the type of residential facilities for children in need of care in Botswana does not fit the typical definition of institutions or orphanages for children. The children's homes mentioned above use a family approach for the care of children. Special effort is made to keep sibling units together (Maundeni, 2009a). The objectives of the residential facilities in Botswana are to create a normal family structure for the children. Members of the

2 These facilities are affiliated to the international organization SOS-Kinderdorf. One village is located in Tlokweng (approximately 4 km from the capital city, Gaborone); the other one is located in Francis town (450 km away from the capital city).

3 It operates from the capital city.

4 Mpule Kwelagobe facility is in Jwaneng (201 km from the capital city).

community are also involved in the care of children in these facilities. Besides meeting basic needs for shelter, food and clothing, the residential facilities also provide psychosocial, spiritual support, healthcare, and enhance the OVC's sense of independence.

An important issue to highlight at this juncture relates to the success of residential facilities as well as their impact on children classified as OVC and their communities. A comprehensive picture of the impact of residential facilities is hard to present given that there is no evidence of evaluation or monitoring in place (Maundeni, 2009b). Similarly, little evidence exists with respect to the success of these institutions. This observation is noteworthy and points to the need for evaluations to determine the effectiveness and other effects of services offered by residential facilities for children in Botswana.

Conclusion

The foregoing discussion has shown that the challenges faced by OVC are enormous. They require innovative responses from all stakeholders. Our discussion also highlighted gaps in addressing the unique challenges faced by children categorized as OVC. We offer recommendations to guide policy and program decisions. Kinship care, as observed, is the most common living arrangement for OVC in Botswana, and we suggest strengthening the capacity of the extended family to effectively protect and care for fostered children. One way to do this would be to introduce programs geared at providing parenting skills as well as emotional and material support. The food basket is an effective example of material support to the needy.

We also learned that children are rarely involved in the decision-making process, even when outcomes have a direct effect on their lives. Mechanisms for the participation of children may need to be put in place at the community and national levels. Schools and other community-based institutions could play a significant role in making this a reality. Another area that may need strengthening is the role of the elderly caregivers. This could be done through the establishment of support groups that will enable them to provide various types of support to each other (Maundeni and Malinga-Musamba, 2013). Overall, NGOs are doing a good job, however, their capacity is often limited by lack of resources. We recommend that the government increase the amount of resources and other supports given to NGOs. Finally, the observed data gaps point to the need for monitoring and evaluation. This has the potential to ensure that the challenges presented by OVC are effectively addressed.

Bibliography

Central Statistics Office (2003). *Household Income and Expenditure Survey (HEIS)*. Government of Botswana, Gaborone.

Deininger, K., Garcia, M. and Subbarao, K. (2003). AIDS-induced orphanhood as a systemic shock: Magnitude, impact, and program interventions in Africa. *World Bank*, 31, 1201–20.

Department of Social Services (2005). *A Report on Provision of Psychosocial Services to Orphans and Vulnerable Children in Botswana: Issues and Challenges*. Ministry of Local Government, DSS.

Foster, G. (2004). Safety nets for children affected by HIV/AIDS in Southern Africa. In Foster, G. and Pharoah, R. (eds), *A Generation at Risk: HIV/AIDS, Vulnerable Children and Security in Southern Africa* (pp. 65–92). Cape Town: Institute of Security Studies.

Government of Botswana (2008a). *National Situation Analysis on Orphans and Vulnerable Children in Botswana*. Gaborone: Ministry of Local Government, Department of Social Services.

Government of Botswana (2008b). *National Guidelines on the Care of Orphans and Vulnerable Children*. Gaborone: Ministry of Local Government, Department of Social Services.

Government of Botswana/UNICEF (2006). *Mid-term Review of the 2003–2007 Country Programme of Cooperation*. Part 1: Global Overview Report February 2006.

Himonga, C.N. (1985). *Family Property Disputes: The Predicament of Women and Children in a Zambian Urban Community*. London: London School of Economic and Political Science.

Hope, K.R. (1996). Growth, unemployment and poverty in Botswana. *Journal of Contemporary African Studies*, 14(1), 53–67.

Jacques, G. (2003). Alien ways or brave new world? Alternative care policy for orphans in Botswana. In Mulinge, M. and Mufune, P. (eds), *Debt Relief Initiatives and Poverty Alleviation: Lessons from Africa*. South Africa: Africa Institute of South Africa.

Lesetedi, G. and Nandi, N. (1995). A demographic and socio-economic profile of women and men in Botswana: A review of summary indicators of population composition and distribution, mortality, migration and economic ability. In *1991 Population and Housing Census Dissemination Seminar* (pp. 176–88). Gaborone: Central Statistics Office.

Maphalala, B.A. (2007). Coping with grief: A case study of orphans in Bobonong Village (Doctoral Dissertation). University of Botswana.

Maundeni, T. (2002). Wife abuse among a sample of divorced women in Botswana: A research note, in *Violence against Women*.

Maundeni, T. (2004). The silent survivors of HIV/AIDS: A quest for comprehensive inclusive strategies in Botswana. In Kasiram, M., Partab, R. and Dano, B. (eds), *HIV/AIDS in Africa: The Not So Silent Presence*. Durban: Print Connection.

Maundeni, T. (2006). *The Silent Survivors of HIV/AIDS: A Quest for Comprehensive and Inclusive Strategies in Botswana*. Durban.

Maundeni, T. (2009). Care for children in Botswana: The social work role. *Social Work and Society*, 7(1), 13–27.

Maundeni, T. (2009). Residential care for children in Botswana: The past, the present, and the future. In Courtney, M.E. and Iwaniec, D. (eds), *Residential Care for Children: Comparative Perspectives*. New York: Oxford University Press.

Maundeni, T. and Levers, L. (2005). Concerns about child subject research in Botswana: A call for establishing structures and guidelines that protect children and Levers. Paper Presented at the Department of Social Work Seminar, September, 2004.

Maundeni, T. and Malinga-Musamba, T. (2013). The role of informal caregivers in the wellbeing of orphans in Botswana: A literature review. *Child and Family Social Work*, 18, 107–16.

Ministry of Health (2002). *Botswana HIV and AIDS Second Medium Term Plan 1997–2002 (MTPII)*. Gaborone.

Ministry of Local Government (1999). *Short Term Plan of Action on Care of Orphans in Botswana, 1999–2001*. Gaborone: Author.

Ministry of Local Government (2001). *Initial Report to the United Nations Committee for the Convention on the Rights of the Child*. Gaborone: Government Printer.

Moatshe, B. (2004). The impact of declining donor support on the sustainability of non-governmental organizations in Botswana: Insights from some NGO managers in Botswana (Bachelor Thesis). University of Botswana.

Molokomme, A. (1987). The mosaic of Botswana maintenance law. *Botswana Notes and Records*, 19, 129–35.

Ndulo, M. (1984). Widows Under Zambian Law and the Response of the Courts. (Unpublished).

Osei-Hwedie, K. (2000). Orphan care in Botswana: Issues, challenges and prospects. The Orphan Care Programme Workshop, Botswana.

Raditedu, B.L. (2004). Psychosocial impact of orphan-hood on the girl-child: A study of Kalkfotein (Bachelor Thesis). University of Botswana.

Republic of Botswana (1952). *Adoption Act*. Gaborone: Government Printer.

Republic of Botswana (2004). *Botswana AIDS Impact Survey III (BAIS II) CSO*. Gaborone.

Republic of Botswana (2008). *Botswana AIDS Impact Survey III (BAIS III), Preliminary Results: CSO*. Gaborone.

Republic of Botswana (2009). *Children's Act*. Gaborone: Government Printer.

Schapera, I. (1984). *The Tswana International African Institute*. London: Routledge.

Shaibu, S. (2004). Gender, health and ageing. In Machacha, L. and Letsie, L. (eds), *Report on the Workshop Proceedings on Gender and Ageing*. University of Botswana: Gender Policy and Programme Committee.

Testa, M.F. and Rolock, N. (1999). Professional foster care: A future worth pursuing. *Journal of Child Welfare*, 78(1), 108–24.

UNAIDS (1999). *Children Orphaned by HIV/AIDS: Frontline Responses from Eastern and Southern Africa.* New York: UNICEF Division of Communication.

UNAIDS (2004). *AIDS Epidemic Update, December*. www.unaids.org.

UNAIDS (2005). *AIDS Epidemic Update, December*. www.unaids.org.

UNAIDS and WHO (2004). *Report on the Global AIDS Epidemic.* www.unaids.org.

UNDP (2000). Botswana human development report. http://www.undp.org/content/dam/aplaws/publication/en/publications/hiv-aids/botswana-national-human-development-report--towards-an-aids-free-generation/76.pdf.

UNICEF (2004). *Children on the Brink: A Joint Report of New Orphan Estimates and Framework for Action.* New York: UNAIDS/UNICEF/USAID.

UNICEF (2006). *Caring for Children Affected by HIV and AIDS.* Florence: Innocenti Research Centre.

UNICEF (2007). *A World Fit for Children: Mid-Decade Review*. Botswana Progress Report.

UNICEF (2011). Annual Report. Botswana Country Office. http://www.unicef.org/botswana/BCO__Annual_Report_2011.pdf.

UNICEF (2013). Annual Report 2013. Botswana. http://www.unicef.org/about/annualreport/files/Botswana_COAR_2013.pdf.

UNICEF, UNAIDS, UNFPA and WHO (2009). *Children and AIDS: Fourth Stocktaking Report, 2009*. New York: UNICEF.

United Nations (1989). *United Nations Convention on the Rights of the Child.* Geneva: United Nations.

United Nations (2004). *Botswana: Millennium Development Goals Status Report 2004: Achievements, Future Challenges and Choices*. Republic of Botswana and United Nations.

USAID (2004). *Sub-National Distribution and Situation of Orphans: An Analysis of the President's Emergency Plan for AIDS Relief Focus Countries*. Washington, DC: USAID, Bureau for Africa, Office of Sustainable Development.

USAID (2010a). *A Cost Analysis of Selected Orphans and Vulnerable Children (OVC) Programs in Botswana*. USAID/Health Policy Initiative.

USAID (2010b). *Assessing Implementation of Botswana's Program for Orphans and Vulnerable Children*. USAID/Health Policy Initiative.

Chapter 6

Responding to Orphaned and Vulnerable Children in Kenya

Alex Ochumbo, Protus Lumiti, and Nicholas Syano

Introduction and Background Information

In recent years, Kenya has experienced a notable decline in HIV prevalence. This is attributed, in part, to significant behavioral change and in part to increased access to ART. Indeed, national adult HIV prevalence is estimated to have fallen from 10 percent in the late 1990s to about 6.1 percent in 2013 (CIA, 2013; UNAIDS, 2013). Among children (0–14 years) estimates stand at 190,000. Despite the noted decline, the number of children defined as OVC is relatively high. This may be an indication of the high adult mortality that characterizes the virus at maturity. In fact, there is some data indicating that HIV/AIDS mortality accounts for about 60 percent of Kenya's population of orphans (UNAIDS, 2013; USAIDS, 2013). The challenges experienced by children considered vulnerable are well documented. In this chapter we highlight major responses undertaken to address their plight. Understanding these responses is important for many reasons, including appreciation of policy and service gaps. It also helps to highlight resource constraints. Moreover, Kenya, during the past few years, has been defined as a country in transition, whose government is seeking ways to restructure critical elements of the state, including social welfare. Kenya currently reports a value of 0.54 on the Human Development Index (UNDP, 2014); a summary measure of average achievement in key dimensions of human development: such as life expectancy, being knowledgeable and having a decent standard of living. This context offers a unique opportunity for understanding HIV/AIDS and mitigating its impact on children.

Kenya, like many countries impacted by HIV/AIDS, has been unrelenting in its effort to curb the spread of the virus. Effort, in this regard, has focused on prevention, controlling mother-to-child transmission and sustaining infected individuals. The country has also been at the forefront of efforts to promote the welfare of individuals and households affected by HIV/AIDS, especially children. This endeavor is seen in policies and resources devoted to OVC care. During the past few years, Kenya has introduced and implemented over 60 pieces of legislation on the issue of vulnerability as it relates to children. The pieces of legislation highlighted here, for the most part, are a domestication of internationally sanctioned instruments which the country is a part of. Examples of these include the following:

1. The Children Act;
2. The National Plan of Action on OVC;
3. National Policy on Food Security;
4. The Kenya National HIV and AIDS Strategic Plan;
5. The National Policy on Orphans and Vulnerable Children.

Despite this, the bulk of the burden of OVC care has fallen on familial networks as well as local and international civic organizations. Indeed, evidence on the subject indicates that, currently, there are about 83 civic organizations working with children classified as OVC in the country. Most of these are engaged in the provision of protection against abuse and exploitation, and the provision of psychosocial and material support in the areas of education, food and nutrition services.

The foregoing discussion is suggestive. Multiple entities including communities, government, and civic organizations have taken note of the plight of children classified as OVC. In subsequent sections of this chapter, we review their responses as well as major international instruments that address the needs of children. Our goal is to provide an overview of these and articulate Kenya's performance. This, we hope, will prompt a discussion on how the identified gaps could be addressed.

Global Responses to OVC in Kenya

Kenya is a signatory to numerous international conventions and agreements that provide for the protection of children and promotion of their rights. Among these are the Convention on the Rights of Child (CRC); the Millennium Development Goals, the 1990 World Declaration on the Survival, Protection and Development of Children, which was agreed at the World Summit for Children; the African Charter on the Rights and Welfare of the Child (ACRWC); and the United Nations AIDS Strategy of 2010. In this section we focus only on three: UNAIDS, CRC, and the Millennium Development Goals. The purpose of this review is to present an overview of progress made on major milestones with regards to the welfare of children classified as vulnerable.

The United Nations AIDS Strategy (UNAIDS)

The strategy was spearheaded by the United Nations General Assembly special session on HIV/AIDS which was convened in June 2001. The special session was a response to the death and suffering that the HIV epidemic had caused worldwide. Heads of state and representatives of governments, at this meeting, came together and expressed commitment to combat HIV/AIDS by signing the

Declaration of Commitment on HIV/AIDS (2001). About 189 UN Member States, including Kenya, adopted the Declaration. Despite the fact that the Declaration is not a legally binding document, it is a clear statement that world governments are committed to fighting the HIV epidemic. The Declaration also helped set targets and deadlines on this agenda. It was against this background that, in 2010, the United Nations AIDS Strategy was adopted with the primary goal of revolutionizing HIV prevention, catalyzing treatment, care, and support. With respect to Africa, the strategy focuses on ensuring that the continent achieves zero new HIV infections, zero discrimination and zero AIDS-related deaths by the year 2015. It also aims at advancing human rights and gender equality, especially as these relate to the care and protection of children (UNAIDS, 2013).

Although sub-Saharan Africa is one of the regions severely affected by HIV, recent data reveals that the region has made considerable strides in its response to HIV/AIDS. Indeed, effort to combat the disease is paying off: the region has the second highest access to HIV treatment—about 56 percent of people living with HIV received antiretroviral therapy in 2011. Infected people are living long, productive lives! Effort toward prevention and halting the spread of HIV/AIDS is also promising. Initiatives to prevent mother-to-child transmission have been implemented; awareness raising campaigns have been conducted; programs to encourage abstinence and condom use have also been put in place. In the specific case of Kenya, general prevalence has been in decline for the past two decades (AVERT, 2014; Kenya National Bureau of Statistics, 2010). Indeed, the rate was 6.7 percent in 2003, 7.4 percent in 2007, and is currently estimated to be 6.2 percent.

As previously discussed, although HIV prevalence among the general population has fallen country-wide, women continue to be disproportionately affected by the epidemic. In 2012, 6.9 percent of women were living with HIV compared with 4.2 percent of men (NASCOP, 2012). Young women (aged 15–24) have a higher likelihood of living with HIV than men of the same age (3 percent vs. 1.1 percent). These figures may be explained by the higher likelihood of young women, in Kenya, to be exposed to sexual violence than young men (KNBS, 2010); their probability of being forced into early marriages and inability to negotiate safe sex. In addition, young women tend to have lower levels of HIV knowledge compared to men in the same age category. Existing evidence suggests that only about 47.5 percent of young women could correctly identify ways of preventing sexual transmission of HIV and reject misconceptions about HIV transmission compared to 54.9 percent of young men (KNBS, 2010). A possible explanation for this is that, like in many parts of sub-Saharan Africa, women and girls in Kenya have limited access to education, employment, and healthcare. Mainly because of their subordinate position, men are often dominant in sexual relationships; women are often unlikely to practice safer sex even when they know the risks.

Progress toward achieving set targets with respect to prevention and treatment has been slower than expected. The Kenya National AIDS Strategic Plan (KNASP III) reports that the target of reaching at least 80 percent of those in need of ART is not expected to be achieved by the year 2015. This is partly due to the fact that availability of ART has not kept pace with the increasing demand. The National AIDS and STI Control Program (NASCOP) estimates that only 68 percent of people in need of ART were able to receive the intervention. With regards to prevention, awareness campaigns continue to be conducted in both schools and other public spaces. Moreover, a significant increase has been recorded in condom use. The NACC estimated an increase in condom supply from 28.4 million in 2005 to 36.2 million in 2006 and further to 64.5 million in 2007. Current figures stand at 180 million (IRIN, 2011; UNGASS, 2014).

With regards to OVC care and protection, available data suggest that considerable progress has been made. Roughly 2.5 million children in Kenya are classified as OVC. As noted, historically, households caring for children in this group have received little assistance from the government. Indeed, only about 14 percent of such children received public support of any kind in 2005. In addition, focused support for children orphaned or made vulnerable by AIDS accounted for only a modest share of HIV spending. For example, in 2007–8, such programs represented less than 3 percent of all HIV expenditures (NACC, 2009). In recent years, the proportion of children receiving support from the government has grown to 21.4 percent (NACC, 2010). The observed progress reflects Kenya's dedication to the promise made in the Declaration of Commitment on HIV/AIDS and new national HIV strategy—KNASP III—which set a target of providing public support to about 40 percent of households caring for OVC. Moreover, the government has domesticated major international instruments to enhance national capacity to address the needs of HIV-affected children and the households caring for them. The national policy and action plan for OVC put in place in 2005 are such examples. These policies have facilitated the introduction and expansion of cash transfer programs to households with vulnerable children, development of quality standards for children's services, implementation of child protection systems, and strengthened family-based care for children classified as vulnerable.

Challenges, however, persist with regards to attitudes toward people living with and affected by HIV. Generally, attitudes toward people living with HIV have become increasingly positive country-wide—rising from 27 percent to 33 percent among men, and from 39.4 percent to 47 percent among women between 2003 and 2009. Despite this, levels of stigma and discrimination remain too high to foster an environment for a more effective national HIV response. Indeed, many people living with and affected by HIV still face high levels of stigma and discrimination. In fact, available evidence suggest that fear of stigma and discrimination deter Kenyans living with HIV from seeking vital HIV services (UNGASS, 2014). For example, there is data suggesting that pregnant women are reluctant to test for HIV because they fear stigmatization from their family and/or healthcare workers.

In addition, while the gains made in OVC care are laudable, much more needs to be done to mitigate the epidemic's impact on children orphaned or made vulnerable by AIDS. Nationally, 35 percent of Kenyan children under the age of five experience moderate or severe stunting, pointing to a shortfall in food security (Kenya National Bureau of Statistics, 2010). Nutritional support may be especially needed for children classified as vulnerable. Shelter and safe employment opportunities may need to be provided, especially for children who live on the streets. The community model utilized by Nyumbani Village may serve as a useful starting point.

Kenya and the Convention on the Rights of Children (CRC)

The government of Kenya recognizes the rights of the child as fundamental to national development. Notable among these are the rights enshrined in Articles 22 and 25 of the United Nations Universal Declaration of Human Rights (1948):

> Everyone as a member of society, has a right to social security … [and] to a standard of living adequate for the health and well-being of himself and his family, including food, clothing, housing, medical care and necessary social services.

The rights of the child guaranteed under the CRC have, in fact, been domesticated by Kenya and form the basis for policies and programming for children. The four principles of the CRC are especially relevant to OVC care:

1. The right to survival, development, and protection from abuse and neglect (Art. 6);
2. Non-discrimination (Art. 2);
3. The right to have a voice and be heard (Art. 12);
4. That the best interests of the child should be of primary consideration (Art. 3);

The CRC underscores the importance of these rights by setting non-negotiable standards and obligations in healthcare, education, legal, civil, and social services. The Convention reaffirms the responsibility of the state in the protection of children's rights, without discrimination of any kind and through the adoption of all appropriate legislative, administrative, budgetary, and any other measures that may be necessary.

The government of Kenya has long recognized the rights of its children. As noted earlier, one avenue for this has been domestication of CRC and its basic underpinning in legislation such as the Child Act of 2001. Priority is given to addressing the vulnerabilities faced by children affected by and living with HIV. Guided by this mandate, the government of Kenya has dedicated attention to children orphaned and made vulnerable by HIV/AIDS. One of the areas of focus has been improving the welfare of children through income-generating activities such as cash transfers. The initiative has resulted in enhanced life chances for Kenya's children and has enabled them to come out of a place of deprivation and despair.

The infusion of HIV/AIDS awareness campaigns into the school curriculum has been effective. The campaign has helped prevent new infections by providing children with information about HIV and how it is passed on; equipping them with the knowledge to protect themselves. It has also helped reduce stigma and discrimination. This effort is commendable. However, it may need to be accompanied by effort to protect children from sexual exploitation—especially children in high risk situations.

Furthermore, although Kenya has ratified the CRC and has implemented/adapted various human rights instruments, available data fails to clearly articulate the country's position with respect to the basic principles of the CRC in response to HIV/AIDS. Realization of rights guaranteed under the CRC may be determined by efforts targeting the capacity of households/families and communities to protect and care for their children. Indeed, children are nested in these social structures.

Improving the lives of children classified as vulnerable is both a legal and moral imperative. Data suggests Kenya has made strides in this area through scaling up social protection programs for children. These programs, e.g., cash transfers, advance a promising vision of social justice. They reflect the realization that caring for society's vulnerable members is a collective responsibility to be shared by a country's government, local citizens, and the international community. The main challenge to this may be limited resources. Indeed, only about 9 percent of total HIV spending is devoted to OVC care.

Kenya and the Millennium Development Goals (MDGs)

Another global initiative of relevance to this discussion is the Millennium Development Goals of 2000. We focus the discussion on the three goals which are relevant to the rights of children, including OVC: universal primary education, gender equality in education, and halting and reversing the spread of HIV/AIDS.

Universal primary education

Over the past few years, net primary enrollment in most African countries has grown significantly, with ratios exceeding 90 percent in several countries. Completion rates with respect to primary education, however, have remained low—they are as low as 33 percent in some countries. Dropout rates, typically, tend to be higher among girls than boys. Factors associated with universal primary education are many and consist of teacher absenteeism, age entry by children in primary school, poor health and nutritional status of both the children and caregivers, financial constraints, distance to school, and quality of education.

In the case of Kenya, net primary enrollment has increased considerably since 2002 when the government of Kenya introduced free primary education which enabled children to begin schooling at the appropriate age. Available data indicates an increase of 2.3 percent between 2005 and 2009 in net enrollment. The National Enrolment Rate (NER) has remained relatively stable through the years and now stands at 82 percent. The Gross Enrolment Rate (GER), for the same period, was

109.8 percent and 110 percent (UNDP, 2010). This ratio, however, is relatively higher for boys compared to girls. For example, in 2009, it stood at 113 percent for boys versus 112 percent for their female counterparts. Retention, completion, and progression rates continue to be problematic and pose a concern with respect to the realization of the millennium goal on education. Low completion rates from primary to secondary school may also be a reflection of the quality of primary education in the country.

Table 6.1 Kenya's performance on targeted goals

Goal and target	Indicator for monitoring progress	Kenya's position (2005–13)
Goal 2: Achieve universal primary education	Net enrollment ratio in primary education	88% in 2002 to 115% in 2011
Target: Ensure that children everywhere, boys and girls alike, will be able to complete a full course of primary schooling	Proportion of pupils starting grade 1 who reach last grade of primary	67% in 2009 to 73% in 2011
	Literacy rate of 15–24-year-olds (women and men)	Not available
Goal 3: Promote gender equality and the empowerment of women	Ratios of girls to boys in primary, secondary, and tertiary education	Gender parity attained
Target: Eliminate gender disparity in primary and secondary education, and in all levels of education	Share of women in wage employment in the non-agricultural sector	29.8% in 2011
	Proportion of seats held by women in national parliament	Female MPs at 9.9% in 2011 up from 4.1% in 1998
Goal 6: Combat HIV/AIDS, malaria and other diseases	HIV prevalence among population aged 15–24 years	2.9% in 2011 down from 3.8% in 2007
Target: Have halted by 2015 and begun to reverse the spread of HIV/AIDS	Condom use at last high-risk sex	
	Proportion of population aged 15–24 years with comprehensive correct knowledge of HIV/AIDS	
	Ratio of school attendance of orphans to school attendance of non-orphans aged 10–14 years	

Source: Created using data from UNDP (2010, p. 130).

With regards to literacy rates in sub-Saharan Africa, these remain low at 72 percent for both sexes. As might be expected, female illiteracy rates are higher than men's. Indeed, inadequate numeracy and literacy skills among primary school leavers are not uncommon. In the case of Kenya the rate is estimated to be 87.4 percent (90.6 percent for men and 84.2 percent for women).

Overall, there has been a marked increase in primary enrollment rates in Kenya. However, regional and gender disparities remain, especially in rural areas, areas of high poverty, and urban slums. Further, unlike many parts of sub-Saharan Africa, data from Kenya suggests high levels of school enrollment and attendance by children classified as vulnerable (Bicego et al., 2003; Case et al., 2004; Monasch and Boerma, 2004). Indeed, data from the NACC (2010) indicates that orphans aged 10–14 have the same rate of school attendance as non-orphans.

Gender equality and the empowerment of women

Considerable progress has been made in sub-Saharan Africa with respect to gender parity despite the fact that the region reported the lowest Gender Parity Index (GPI) of 0.92 in 2012. Gender disparities are said to be higher in secondary and tertiary education. This tends to spill over into the labor market, limiting the ownership of productive assets by women. Challenges like poverty, early marriage, and child labor have contributed to the observed trend. In recent years, reforms such as the introduction of free primary education have helped in narrowing the gap.

To curb the observed discrepancies, the government of Kenya has devoted resources targeting social services to improve the welfare of groups considered vulnerable. Specifically, the Ministry of Gender, Children and Social Services recorded the highest increase in expenditure of 82.3 percent from 2002 to 2010. Further, the expenditure of the central government on social services related to gender increased from KES 1,421.42 in 2008/9 to 3,049.36 million in the 2009/10 financial year. In addition, Kenya's current constitution, which was inaugurated in 2010, has provided for 30 percent representation of women in elected and public office (see Table 6.1 for additional data).

An increase of 82.3 percent in gender targeted expenses is remarkable. However, it is not clear how the expenditure has translated into gains for women and children. The data available on the subject suggests that the share of women in wage employment in the non-agricultural sector is about 30 percent. These data also reveal progress in the proportion of seats held by women in national parliament—the number of female members of parliament rose from 4.1 percent in 1998 to 9.9 percent in 2011 (UNDP, 2012).

Combat HIV/AIDS

The HIV outlook for young people (aged 15–24) has also changed positively in sub-Saharan Africa over the years. As observed, young females are more susceptible to HIV infection than males, although females have experienced a sharper decline in prevalence rates (5.1 to 3.1 percent compared with 2.0 to 1.3 percent) over the period 2005 to 2011. Indeed, favorable changes with respect to risky sexual behavior within this age group are evident in many countries, including Kenya (UNAIDS, 2012). Also, condom use is generally on the rise in sub-Saharan Africa. However, awareness remains low in several of the high-prevalence countries, especially among young women. Besides, condom supply remains inadequate.

The Millennium Development Goals and AIDS, generally, have a feedback loop type relationship, with each feeding into the other. Indeed, eradicating AIDS is essential for achievement of the Millennium Development Goals. On the other hand, progress toward realization of the Millennium Development Goals is crucial to the attainment of the goals of HIV prevention, treatment, care, and support (UNAIDS, 2013). This observation is suggestive; attainment of the MDGs will require a multifaceted effort. Investment in quality education and improving accessibility of schools is a key component of this effort. Another component of this could be upgrading the skills of teachers and encouraging timely entry into school. In addition, consideration could be given to introducing legislation favorable to women and children—e.g., legislation against early marriages. This has potential to improve access to education, reduce dropout rates, and enhance the overall quality of education. Alongside these initiatives, should be effort directed at scaling up prevention and treatment of HIV as well as care for affected individuals, especially children.

Local Responses to OVC

Policy Responses

The response of the Kenyan government to the HIV/AIDS pandemic has been overarching and includes the launch of poster campaigns to raise nationwide awareness (NASCOP, 1987), declaration of the AIDS epidemic as a national disaster, establishment of a National AIDS Control Council, as well implementation of policies and initiatives to help curb the pandemic (AVERT, 2014; Mwaura, 2009; UNGASS, 2006). In fact, in Kenya AIDS education is part of the curriculum in both primary and secondary schools, and for a number of years Kenya has delivered educational campaigns on the issue. This section provides an overview of the following initiatives:

1. The Children Act of 2001;
2. National Policy on Orphans and Vulnerable Children of 2005;
3. National Plan of Action on Orphans and Vulnerable Children (2007–10).

The Children Act of 2001

The Children Act was enacted in 2001 and came into force in March 2002. The Act, which is under the custody of the Ministry of Gender, Children's Services and Social Development, is seen as the most important legislation for children (Odongo, 2004). It provides wide-ranging safeguards for the rights and welfare of the child. It also defines duties and responsibilities of the child-right holder as well as identifying the duty bearers and their responsibilities/obligations to the child (Odongo, 2012). Specifically, the Act facilitates the establishment of the National Council for Children Services (NCC)—which is the main coordinating and unifying agency for children services in the country—enables the establishment of children's courts as well as other services aimed at protecting and promoting the best interest of the child. The Act draws from various local and international instruments and agreements on the protection of children and promotion of their rights that Kenya has adapted. The Act, in a sense, ensures that children in Kenya have an opportunity of realizing their full potential by growing in a safe and stable environment. In particular, it makes provision for parental responsibility, fostering, adoption, custody, maintenance, guardianship, care, and protection of children. It also gives guidance with respect to the administration of children's institutions, gives effect to the principles of the Convention on the Rights of the Child and the African Charter on the Rights and Welfare of the Child.

Since its implementation, the Act, which is the primary legal recognition of the rights of children in Kenyan law, has accomplished many things. For examples, the government estimates that 62 percent of children have birth registration documents. The provision of free primary education (FPE) is associated with an increase in net school enrollment. Furthermore, children classified as vulnerable have been beneficiaries of social programs such as conditional income transfers. Additionally, starting from 2006, three child-specific courts with physically separate court houses and infrastructure designed for children—whether as victims of crimes, witnesses, in need of care and protection, and in conflict with the law—have been established. Also, the provisions of the Child Offender Rules articulated in the Children's Act has been taken into consideration in a number of cases involving children. The provision relates to time limits for trials and the pre-trial detention of children in conflict with the law.

Despite the observed gains, a number of challenges remain. Public ignorance on the importance of birth registration continues to pose as barriers to the registration of births. Inadequacies in registration of births are also connected to insufficient infrastructure. Indeed, only about 40 percent of births took place in health facilities in 2003. This figure has remained relatively unchanged over the years. Moreover, registration of birth is not fully decentralized; families have to travel long distances, particularly in rural areas, to access registration services. The birth notification process is riddled with bureaucracies and may take a year or two to complete.

Furthermore, the Act does not adequately address the rights of children with respect to social security and provisions which spell out the state's obligations in this regard. This is directly connected to the high levels of poverty among children—especially OVC and children who live and work on the street. It is important to note that Kenya has an extraordinarily high number of street children with conservative estimates putting the number at between 250,000 and 300,000

(UNICEF, 2013). Limited capacity of primary duty bearers including parents and other caregivers also present another challenge.

Although the provision of FPE has enabled many children from poor households to attend primary school, problems exist with regards to the girl-child. A significant number of these are likely to drop out of school. Regional variations are evident in school enrollment with poor regions reporting poorer outcomes. Children, for the most part, continue to be under-represented in the decision-making process.

Overall, the Act demonstrates commitment to Kenya's children. It ensures that the rights of children in Kenya are part of policy discussion/s. Most importantly, the Act safeguards the best interest of children in Kenya and offers them an opportunity realize their full potential by growing in a safe and stable environment. Full realization of the rights guaranteed under the Children's Act will require active participation of all the key stakeholders, including children classified as vulnerable. Areas that might need attention include the following:

1. sensitization of the general public;
2. training of professionals;
3. budgeting for children's rights at all levels of government (national, regional, and local);
4. procedural reform within state institutions requiring innovation and dedication of different officials in the implementation process.

National Policy on Orphans and Vulnerable Children of 2005

The initiative was put in place by the National Steering Committee (NSC) on Orphans and Vulnerable Children. The Department of Children Services, within the Ministry of Gender, Children and Social Development, in collaboration with the National Steering Committee on OVC developed the OVC Policy. Its scope of coverage consists of children defined as orphaned (maternal, paternal, and double orphans) and vulnerable. The policy therefore utilizes priority targeting in service delivery (Figure 6.1 presents target groups).

The policy is intended to ensure that every Kenyan child who is orphaned or vulnerable is protected and supported in order to achieve their full potential (Kenya National Policy on Orphaned and Vulnerable Children, 2005). Specifically, the policy seeks to support and protect the rights of OVC in the areas of child survival, child development, child protection, and child participation. Following are its primary objectives:

1. Ensure that orphans and vulnerable children attain their basic survival needs;
2. Support orphans and vulnerable children to develop to their full potential;
3. Protect orphans and vulnerable children from all forms of abuse, exploitation, and discrimination;
4. Ensure the full and meaningful participation of orphans and vulnerable children in all matters affecting their lives.

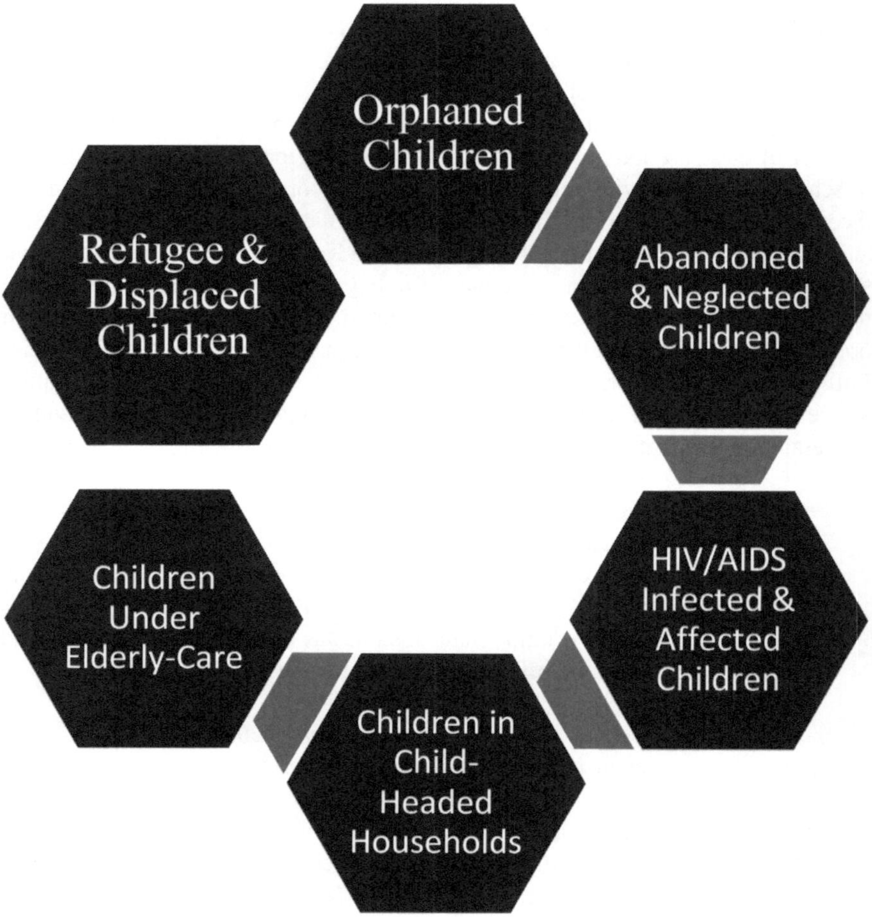

Figure 6.1 Policy target groups
Source: Created using the review—overall.

It is important to note that the implementation of the National Policy on OVC requires that all stakeholders be involved at all levels. Therefore, the policy encourages collaboration and networking among major stakeholders in order to achieve the specified goals—that OVCs in Kenya may be protected and realize their full potential. Since its implementation, gains have been made in areas such as attainment of basic needs. Key aspects of this consist of provision of a regular cash subsidy of about KSH 1,500 per month to households caring for OVC. Cash transfer programs have ensured that OVC are not only enrolled in but also complete basic education. Success has been recorded in facilitating the protection of children defined as OVC. Initiatives that focus on income-generating and livelihood-enhancing opportunities have been implemented as well.

Data scarcities limit meaningful examination in areas such as development of full potential and children's participation. This observation is explained, in part, by the lack of research on this subject and in part by the limited attention devoted to the subject. Indeed, development of full potential seems to be an abstract term, which may not be easy to measure. Capturing participation of children in decision-making may be difficult to access in that this is not a behavior that is endorsed in many of the cultures of sub-Saharan Africa.

The government of Kenya has provided leadership in OVC responses. Policies and guidelines/strategic framework have been put in place. However, the implementation of these, along with the training of staff, has been problematic. In addition, dissemination of the information to the grassroots has been challenging. Also, there is some disconnect between policy provisions across the country. For example in the education sector, policy provisions for school feeding and shelter interventions are largely absent. Further, implementation of the bursary provision for OVC to attend secondary schools has only reached a small proportion of targeted children. Similarly, initiation of flexible schooling options and reviewing school attendance requirements, such as uniforms, which is provided for under the policy, has yet to be implemented. The general assumption has been that the cash transfer program would cater for all OVC needs and requirements. Apart from this, limited awareness of the policy prevails country-wide. Participation of children in both decision-making and programming remains limited. Changing this may require consolidated effort ensuring implementation of mechanisms for listening to the voices of OVC and building their capacity for self-advocacy.

National Plan of Action on OVC (2007–10)

The Department of Children Services, within the Ministry of Gender, Children and Social Development, in collaboration with the National Steering Committee on OVC, played a major role in implementation of the Nation Plan of Action (NPA) for OVC. The primary objective of the NPA is to strengthen the capacity of families to protect and care for OVC as well as mobilize and support community-based responses to OVC. The NPA also presents an avenue for Kenya to realize the milestone articulated in the MDGs with respect to children. Target areas consist of enhancing OVC's access to essential services such as food and nutrition, education, healthcare, housing, water, and sanitation. The NPA further defines and establishes the minimum requirement for OVC care. Specifically, it sets out resources needed for the care of OCV in different age groups and estimates the cost of each component of the minimum requirement (Table 6.2 provides a list of the minimum requirements). It also lays out coordination mechanisms and provides a general outline with regards to monitoring and evaluation. It further presents funding mechanisms for OVC care along with procedures with potential to promote transparency, accountability, and a wider reach of OVC.

While the Department of Children Services plays a major role in supervising OVC interventions in the country, the NPA recognizes that collaboration with other government ministries/departments that provide services for OVC is crucial.

In addition, it affirms the role of civil society, community-based organizations (CBOs), and faith-based organizations (FBOs) as essential partners in addressing OVC needs.

Support given ranges from cash transfers provided by the Department of Children Services, within the Ministry of Gender, Children and Social Development, to the provision of basic necessities along with other forms of social support. These services/interventions have helped stabilize the financial status of families, enhanced skills in small business management, strengthened life and survival skills, provided psychosocial support, bed-nets, clothes, shoes, and bedding to children and their families. Another component of this is the provision of free ART to HIV-infected people. This has enabled many infected individuals, including children, to live longer. Additionally, the NPA has enabled communities to provide support to children in child-headed households. It has also made provision of protection of vulnerable children a priority across many parts of Kenya. Support, in addition, has been provided to caregivers, especially older adults and grandparents, caring for children.

Overall, gains have been made through the NPA. Challenges remain in many areas, including participation, coordination, and lack of evidence to guide policy and program decisions. Data available indicates lack of participation of children including OVC in NPAs across sub-Saharan Africa. This is troubling for many reasons, including the fact that children understand their needs and hence are better positioned to articulate them. Furthermore, rights and requirements for care differ across age groups. For example, mainly because young children require more caregiving and are less able to help with household chores and other work than older children, they may be perceived as a greater burden to overworked caregivers. There is also the issue of protection from poor treatment, stigma, or loss of rights. Participation and voice is part of the rights guaranteed to children under both the CRC and the Children's Act.

With regards to coordination, this is essential in that it reduces replication and allows for effective resource management. Effort is therefore needed to strengthen structures for networking and coordination at the local, regional, and national levels. Alongside this, is the need for research or evidence on the magnitude of the problem, its effects on children as well as effectiveness of interventions put in place in response to problems experienced by OVC and their caregivers. Attention to this will ensure more effective responses. It may provide accurate information on the magnitude of the problem. There is some evidence suggesting that a substantial number of young children who are orphans and/or vulnerable tend to escape notice; they often fall through the cracks. Furthermore, the exercise may produce knowledge on nutrition, health, sanitation, and psychosocial support that may not be available to grandparents or other alternate caregivers.

Table 6.2 List of minimum requirements

Service category	Provision
Education	Allows for provision of school fees, uniforms, books, and other school related needs/supplies.
Health and nutrition	Provides resources required for a full course of immunization, vitamin supplements, and routine healthcare services for children aged 0–5 years. Provides resources to cover routine healthcare services for children aged 6–17 years. Increase the accessibility and quality of healthcare for children Providing nutritional food supplements for young children.
Social services	Enables birth registration for children aged 0–5 years and those aged 6–17 who were not registered at birth or early childhood. Psychosocial support to both children and their caregivers.
Vocational training	Provides training for OVC who may not wish to continue with formal schooling. Capacity building.

Source: Created using data from National Plan of Action for Orphans and Vulnerable Children Kenya (2008, p. 138).

Responses from Community-Based Organizations

With limited public sector support in the past for initiatives to mitigate the epidemic's impact on children, development partners, civil society groups, and community-based organizations have worked closely with affected households and communities to close the gaps in access to needed assistance. Current estimates are that there are approximately 2,100 registered NGOs and community-based organizations in Kenya. Although the exact number of organizations working on OVC in Kenya is not known, existing data indicates that the Kenya AIDS NGO Consortium (KANCO) has about 800 member organizations with funding from USAID. Most of the care is provided by non-governmental organizations, followed by community-based organizations as well as private not-for-profit agencies and the government.

Care strategies include mobilization and training of community-based organizations in OVC care, raising awareness of the needs of children, along with provision of psychosocial support. A comprehensive list of these is provided in Table 6.3.

Table 6.3 Categories of OVC care

Services provided
Advocacy and awareness raising campaigns
Capacity building and community mobilization
Education and vocation training
Food and nutrition services
Protection against abuse and exploitation
Psychosocial support

Source: Created using data from National Plan of Action for Orphans and Vulnerable Children Kenya (2008, p. 139).

Non-governmental organizations have been the primary drivers in OVC care. What may be needed is effort directed at monitoring and evaluation with a focus on program outcomes. Indeed, the evidence currently in place has focused mainly on capturing the number of children served or services provided. Data on numbers of OVC, program impact, and program cost appear to be missing in the current OVC evidence base. The lack of information tends to hinder implementation of evidence-based policy and program decisions. This picture, however, is not likely to change given the limited resources available to split between programming and research. Enhancing networking between OVC programs for data sharing and quality of care and service delivery may be important.

The effects of the HIV/AIDS epidemic on children in Kenya, like any country in sub-Saharan Africa, are manifold; thousands of children are infected with HIV, and most are left undiagnosed, do not have access to treatment, and often die very young. Others are HIV/AIDS affected and have their life chances highly compromised. A combination of factors can improve the situation. Evidence suggests that greater access to mother-to-child transmission prevention interventions, appropriate testing, efficient linkages to care and treatment, as well as support to families and communities have been effective. Intensified efforts may be needed to enhance coordination, harmonization, and alignment of the national response so they meet the needs of impacted children effectively. It is evident that progress has been made in the last 30 years, yet more is needed, especially with regards to strengthening the country's healthcare system. Finally, families, friends, and the wider community have been the first line of protection and support for children classified as OVC. They have provided for their material as well as social, psychological, and emotional needs. Supporting a family holistically may be the best way to ensure quality of life for the child. Social protection schemes that provide external assistance to poor families in areas where HIV prevalence is high may be a viable way of improving the lives of children affected by AIDS. Children benefit from better nutrition, the opportunity to go to school instead of work, and better access to healthcare when a household's economic burden is reduced. Moreover, children benefit from the emotional support that is provided through the family.

Bibliography

AVERT: AVERTing HIV and AIDS (2014). HIV and AIDS in Kenya. www.avert.org/hiv-aids-kenya.htm.

Bicego, G., Rutstein, S., and Johnson, K. (2003). Dimensions of the emerging orphan crisis in sub-Saharan Africa. *Social Science and Medicine*, 56(6): 1235–47.

Care Kenya (2004). *A Baseline Study on the Situation of Orphans and Vulnerable Children (OVC) in Kibera.*

Care Kenya (2007). *A Study on the Violation of the Legal Rights of OVC, Vulnerable Women and People Living with HIV/AIDS.*

Case, A., Paxson, C., and Ableidinger. J. (2004). Orphans in Africa: Parental death, poverty, and school enrollment. *Demography*, 41(3): 483–508.

Central Intelligence Agency (CIA) (2013). *The World Factbook 2013–2014.* Washington, DC: Author.

Gaciuki, P. (2005). Child headed households the emerging phenomenon in urban informal settlements: A case study of Kibera slum Nairobi Kenya. Unpublished MA project paper, University of Nairobi.

Human Rights Watch (2001). *In the Shadow of Death: HIV/AIDS and Children's Rights in Kenya*, 13(4): (A).

IRIN (2011). Zimbabwe: Cash transfers target vulnerable children. http://newirin.irinnews.org/.

KAACR (2003). An assessment of the implementation of the Children Act in Courts KAIS Collaborating Institutions (2009, September) "Kenya AIDS Indicator Survey 2007."

Kenya National Bureau of Statistics (KNBS) and ICF Macro (2010). *Kenya Demographic and Health Survey 2008–09*. Calverton: KNBS and ICF Macro.

Kenya National Policy on Orphaned and Vulnerable Children (KNPOVC) (2005). Republic of Kenya. Nairobi, Kenya: Office of the Vice-President and Ministry of Home Affairs.

Monasch, R. and Boerma, J.T. (2004). Orphanhood and childcare patterns in sub-Saharan Africa: An analysis of national surveys from 40 countries. *AIDS*, 18: S55–S65.

Moody, B. (2007). AIDS leaves Africa's grannies to raise children. Reuters, November 28. http://www.reuters.com/article/idUSL27480920071128?pageNumber=2andvirtualBrandChannel=0andsp=true.

Mwaura, E. (2009). HIV/AIDS Prevention Strategies in Kenya. A critical review. Master's Thesis, University of Pittsburgh.

NACC (2009). *Kenya National AIDS Spending Assessment: Report for the Financial Years 2006/07 and 2007/08*. Nairobi: Author.

NACC (2010). *UNGASS 2010: United Nations General Assembly Special Session on HIV and AIDS Country Report—Kenya*. Nairobi: Author.

NACC (2014). *Kenya AIDS Response Progress Report 2014: Progress towards Zero*. Nairobi: Author.

NASCOP (1987). *Kenya AIDS Newsletter*. Nairobi: Author.

NASCOP (2006). *UNGASS 2006: United Nations General Assembly Special Session on HIV and AIDS Country Report—Kenya*. Nairobi: Author.

NASCOP (2012). *The Kenya AIDS Epidemic UPDATE 2011*. Nairobi: Author.

National Plan of Action for Orphans and Vulnerable Children Kenya 2007–2010 (NPAOVC) (2008). Nairobi, Kenya: Department of Children Services.

Odongo, G. (2012). Caught between progress, stagnation and a reversal of some gains: Reflections on Kenya's record in implementing children's rights norms. *African Human Rights Law Journal*, 12(1): 112–41.

Odongo, G.O. (2004). The domestication of international standards on the rights of the child: A critical and comparative evaluation of the Kenyan example. *The International Journal of Children s Rights*, 12(4): 419–30.

Office of the Vice-President and Ministry of Home Affairs (2005). *National Policy on Orphans and Vulnerable Children Draft 3: 07.05.05*. Nairobi: Author.

UNAIDS (2012). *Global Report: UNAIDS Report on the Global AIDS Epidemic 2012*. Geneva: Author.

UNAIDS (2013). *Global Report: UNAIDS Report on the Global AIDS Epidemic 2013*. Geneva: Author.

UNAIDS, UNICEF and USAID (2002). Children on the Brink 2002: A Joint Report on Orphan Estimates and Program Strategies. Washington, DC: TvT Associates. www.usaid.gov and http://www.unicef.org/media/publications/children_on_brink.pdf.

UNDP (2010). *Kenya National Human Development Report 2009*. Nairobi: UNDP Kenya.

UNDP (2012). Working towards sustainable development: 2012 annual report and financial statements. http://www.ke.undp.org/content/kenya/en/home/library/annual-reports/undp-kenya-annual-report-20120/.

UNDP (2014). Human development report: Human development index. http://www.undp.org/content/undp/en/home/presscenter/events/2014/july/HDR2014.html.

Undugu Society of Kenya (2007). The incidence/prevalence of glue sniffing and any other inhalants among children and vulnerable youth living and working in the streets of Nairobi.

UNGASS (2006). Country progress report—Kenya.

UNGASS (2014). Kenya AIDS Response Progress report: progress towards zero. National AIDS Control Council. http://www.unaids.org/sites/default/files/country/documents/KEN_narrative_report_2014.pdf.

UNICEF (1999). *Children Orphaned by AIDS: Front-Line Responses from Eastern and Southern Africa*. New York: UNICEF.

UNICEF (2006). Extent and effect of sex tourism and sexual exploitation of children on the Kenyan coast. A study conducted by UNICEF and the Government of Kenya.

UNICEF (2013). Annual Report—Kenya. http://www.unicef.org/about/annualreport/files/Kenya_COAR_2013.pdf.

UNICEF and UNAIDS (2010). *Children and AIDS Seventh Stocktaking Report.* http://www.unicef.org/publications/index_57005.html.

USAID (2013). Kenya 2013 report of the people: The US-Kenya partnership. https://www.usaid.gov/sites/default/files/documents/1860/USAID%20Kenya%202013%20Annual%20Report.pdf.

Chapter 7
Responding to Orphaned and Vulnerable Children in Zambia

Theresa Lungu, Chrisann Newransky, and Aakanksha Sinha

Magnitude of the OVC Phenomenon in Zambia

The number of orphans and vulnerable children (OVC) in Zambia has been on the increase since the 1990s (CSO, 2009; Republic of Zambia, 2010). Current estimates are that about 60 percent of all children in Zambia are OVC. A significant proportion of these have suffered the loss of a parent/s (about 49 percent) due to HIV and AIDS (Republic of Zambia, 2010; UNGASS, 2011). This number includes about 13 to 27 percent of all children below the age of 15 (Living Conditions Monitoring Survey, 2006; UNGASS, 2011). Further, about 19 percent of OVC in the country are double orphans, a group particularly vulnerable compared to children who have at least one parent living (National AIDS Council, 2012; Zambia Demographic Health Survey, 2013–14).

It is important to note that the incidence of HIV in adults aged 25–49 years in Zambia has halved since 1990 and was estimated to be at a stable level at 1.6 percent in 2009 (2 percent in women, 1.2 percent in men). Also, the number of new infections among children aged 0–14 years has gone down dramatically since its peak level of 21,189 in 1996 (ZHDR, 2007). However, the number of children made vulnerable by HIV/AIDS related factors has been on the rise since 2004—growing by 13 percent from 2004 to 2008 (Malcom, 2009; MOE Census, 2009; UNGASS, 2011). Reports from UNICEF suggest that there are 226 new adult infections and 25 new child infections that occur each day (UNICEF, 2013). In fact, current estimates suggest that this figure is likely to rise significantly as the epidemic matures and adult AIDS mortality rates increase.

Recent estimates are that the population of OVC in sub-Saharan Africa is fairly young—about 30 percent are aged between 6 and 10, while 18 percent are under the age of 5 (Hutchinson et al., 2009; UNICEF, 2008). The mean age of OVC in the region is estimated to be 6.2 years (Mugabe et al., 2002). In the case of Zambia, while a fair amount of data exists on OVC, there is a dearth of data that accurately reflect the demographic characteristics of this group. Available data suggest that boys make up about 45 percent of OVC. The average age ranges from 9.6 to 12.2 (UNGASS, 2011). Furthermore, compared to children in rural localities, urban children are more likely to be orphaned or vulnerable (16 percent vs. 27 percent). Another factor of note with regards to OVC in Zambia is the bias in delivery of services for OVC, which seems to favor urban areas because the majority of public, private, and civil society organizations are located in these areas (National AIDS Council, 2012; Center for Global Health & Development Boston University, 2010).

Overview of Responses to OVC

Historically, the familial system has provided care to orphaned and vulnerable children. The general expectation has been that when a family experiences loss of one or two parents, the extended family will absorb surviving children. In certain cases, e.g., when surviving members of the extended family lack resources, the community may step in to help in the care of orphaned children. Faith-based organizations have also provided support to OVC. Government, through customary law, has been involved in the care of women and children (upon the death of a breadwinner) by laying out inheritance rights. However, customary law does not have a provision on inheritance rights by children; nor does it provide guidelines for the care of OVC by the extended family.

A legal framework for addressing the needs of OVC in Zambia has been put in place during the past few years. This encompasses policies and guidelines aimed at strengthening care and support structures for OVC. The framework also stipulates measures to promote and support community-based care of OVC. Primary among these are the National Child Policy of 2006, Public Welfare Assistance Schemes, and the National HIV and AIDS Strategic Framework (Republic of Zambia, 2010). Moreover, the country's commitment to the survival, wellbeing, and development of vulnerable children is expressed in ratification of international treaties such as the Convention on the Rights of the Child, the African Charter, the Millennium Development Goals, and the UN Declaration of Commitment on HIV/AIDS "Global Crisis—Global Action" (Republic of Zambia, 2010; UNGASS, 2010, 2011).

Non-governmental organizations, to a large extent, have played a major role in the care of OVC. Their effort extends from service delivery to building and strengthening community capacity (UNICEF, 2005). The burden of caring for OVC, generally, leans heavily on the extended family and local communities. Women, especially the elderly (aged grandparents for the most part), shoulder the responsibility for fostering and providing psychosocial support at the household level. This is especially the case for double orphans. In short, responses to OVC in Zambia are best understood through two lenses: the formal, encompassing provisions from governmental and non-governmental organizations; and the informal, comprising mainly of familial and community-based support.

Governmental Response to the Needs of OVC in Zambia

Responses to the needs of OVC in Zambia are deeply rooted in the African philosophical orientation of Convivencia or Ubuntuism—the idea that we are interconnected by virtue of our shared humanity. From this background, a child is valued, protected, and cared for because she belongs to the greater whole—society. There is also the belief that the greater whole is diminished when others, especially its weaker/vulnerable members, are deprived, stigmatized, humiliated, and/or dehumanized. Tied to this is the view that "children are the future" of any human society and communal responsibility for the welfare of children.

As is the case in most of sub-Saharan Africa, HIV/AIDS has resulted in a rapidly growing population of OVC, threatening the survival, growth, and development of children in this group (UNICEF, 2008). Consequently, the capacity of the traditional safety net provided by the extended family has been severely strained, challenging the social fabric and the concept of "Ubuntu" upon which Zambian society is built (Chatterji et al., 2010; Wallis et al., 2010). Government has been forced to act, to help fill the void left by the traditional systems of care and provide about 30 percent of the total OVC services nationwide (tables 7.1 and 7.2 provide an overview of types of services provided by the government and costs by service domain). For the most part, therefore, the evolution of formal responses to OVC has not been innate and systematic—it has been convoluted; necessitated by the vast needs presented by OVC. Major international treaties have also been a factor in shaping responses to OVC. An overview of these is presented in subsequent sections.

Table 7.1 Types of OVC services provided by government

Service provided	No. of districts covered (N = 72)	Service provider (gov't ministry or agency)
Institutional care	4	MSYCD
Temporary housing/foster care	8	MCDSS
Birth registration and birth certificates	12	MSYCD
Day-care/nursery	14	MCDSS
Vocational training and/or income-generating activities	16	MCDSS
Access to legal protection	19	MSYCD
Registering orphaned children	20	MSYCD
Provision of food basket	22	MCDSS
Health related services	24	Ministry of Health/ MCDSS
Youth clubs	25	MCDSS
Material support/personal care	26	MCDSS
Education support	27	MCDSS
Psychosocial support/counseling	30	MCDSS
Social protection/cash transfers	13	MCDSS

Note: MSYCD = Ministry of Sport, Youth and Child Development; MCDSS = Ministry of Community Development and Social Services.
Source: Created using data from the National AIDS Council (2012, p. 146).

Table 7.2 Cost of government services provided to OVC by service domain

Service area	Total costs (in BWP)	Total cost (in USD)	Percentage
Food and nutrition	33,307,535	4,766,308	61
Education	10,658,807	1,525,275	20
Shelter and care	7,292,320	1,043,531	13
Clothing and bedding	2,767,848	396,079	5
Psychological support	640,278	91,624	1

Source: Created using data from Health and Development and Health and Development Africa (2010) and UNGASS (2010, p. 146).

International Treaties and Children in Zambia

The government of Zambia is a signatory to, and has ratified, major international treaties and conventions with respect to the child. Primary among these are the Convention on the Rights of the Child (CRC), the African Charter on the Rights of the Child (ACRWC), and the Millennium Development Goals (MDGs). The Zambian government is also party to the United Nations General Assembly 26th Special Session (UNGASS) on the Declaration of Commitment on HIV/AIDS. In this section we review international instruments/treaties and examine how these have shaped the government's response to the plight of OVC in the country.

Convention on the Rights of the Child

The Convention on the Rights of the Child is the first legally binding international instrument to incorporate the full range of human rights—civil, cultural, economic, political, and social rights—as they pertain to children. The Convention sets out these rights in 54 articles and two optional protocols. It spells out the basic human rights that children everywhere have: the right to survival; to develop to the fullest; to protection from harmful influences, abuse, and exploitation; and to participate fully in family, cultural, and social life (ACPF, 2011). The four core principles of the Convention are non-discrimination; devotion to the best interests of the child; the right to life, survival, and development; and respect for the views of the child (see Figure 7.1). The goal is to promote child-centered policies and programs.

By ratifying or acceding to the Convention in 1991, the Zambian government committed itself to protect and guarantee human rights as they pertain to children. The government, in effect agreed to hold itself accountable to this commitment before the people of Zambia and the international community. States party to the Convention are also obliged to develop and undertake all actions necessary to safeguard the best interest of the child. In this discussion we focus specifically on Articles 25–29 which address health, welfare, and education rights (see Table 7.3).

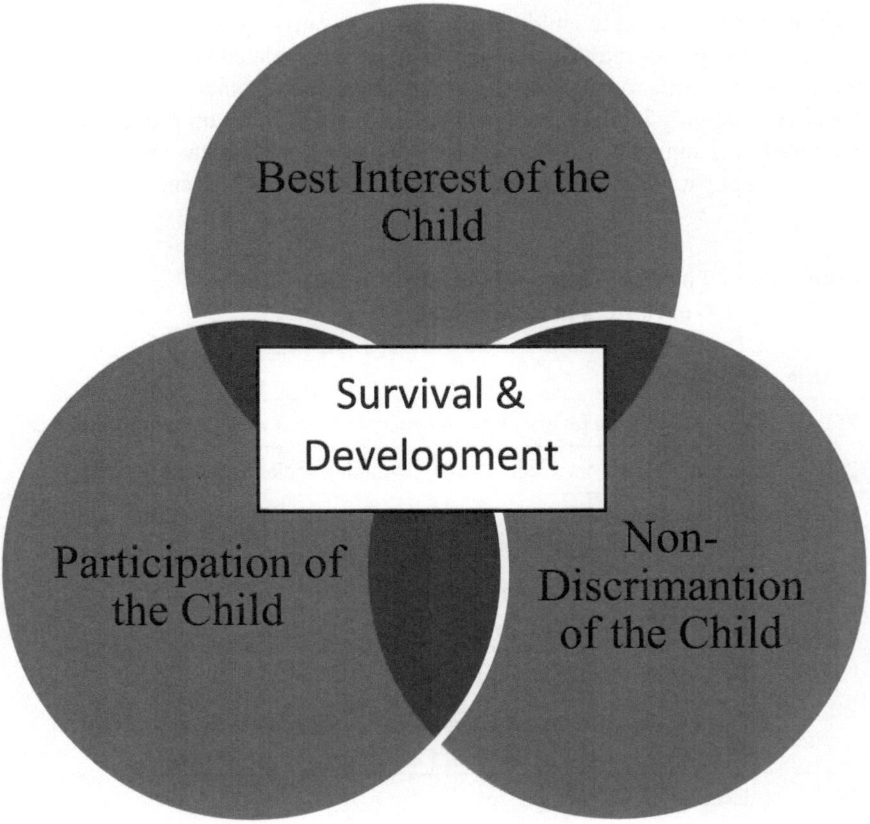

Figure 7.1 Child-centered approaches
Source: Model developed from UNDP's rights-based approaches.

Following ratification of the Convention on the Right of the Child, a number of provisions have been incorporated into national laws. For example, the government has outlawed the corporal punishment of children and introduced stiffer penalties on defilement and trafficking of children. Zambia has also strengthened its commitment to availing universal primary education and access to healthcare (National AIDS Council, 2012). The government has also put in place a child policy and established a child and youth parliament along with a youth media. Milestones have been realized with respect to education—safety nets promoting school enrollment and attendance among vulnerable children have been put in place, e.g., waiving of user fees for vulnerable children. Further, a mechanism for the provision of social support has been established in the form of cash transfers. Recently a policy on child labor has been developed, but has not yet been adopted. Despite these policies and programs, challenges still remain. Among these are lack of a clear legal definition of a child, weakly developed system of legislation with respect to children, and failure to ratify optional protocols. There is also a lack of concrete national and local policies related to child welfare and protection, affecting localization and comprehensive implementation of the CRC. Measures currently in place, for the most part, tend to focus on provision of food and nutritional supports. Most importantly, interventions that have been employed have not kept pace with the growing needs of vulnerable children.

Table 7.3 The Convention on the Rights of the Child: Guarantees in each article

Article	Description
25	Right to a periodic review of the treatment of a child who has been placed in care
26	Right to benefit from social security, including social insurance
27	Right to a standard of living adequate for a child's physical, mental, spiritual, moral, and social development
28	Right of the child to education Ensuring that school discipline is administered in a manner consistent with the child's human dignity Promoting and encouraging international cooperation in matters relating to education
29	Education shall be directed to: (a) Developing child's personality, talents and mental and physical abilities to their fullest potential. (b) Respect for human rights and fundamental freedoms. (c) Respect for the child's parents, his or her own cultural identity, language and values, for the national values of the country in which the child is living, the country from which he or she may originate, and for civilizations different from his or her own. (d) Preparing the child for responsible life in a free society, in the spirit of understanding, peace, tolerance, equality of sexes, and friendship among all peoples, ethnic, national and religious groups, and persons of indigenous origin. (e) Respect for the natural environment.

Source: Created using data from UNICEF: http://www.unicef.org/crc/ (p. 148).

The African Charter on the Rights of a Child (ACRWC)

The African Charter on the Rights and Welfare of the Child (also referred to as the Children's Charter) was adopted by the Organization of African Unity (OAU), now the African Union,[1] in 1990 and was entered into force in 1999. Like the United Nations Convention on the Rights of the Child (CRC), the Children's Charter is a comprehensive instrument that spells out rights in relation to children and defines principles and norms with respect to children in Africa. The Children's Charter also covers a spectrum of civil, political, economic, social, and cultural rights. Why is there a need for the Children's Charter, one might ask? This instrument was created in response to concerns expressed by member states of the African Union (African Committee of Experts on the Rights of the Child, n.d.) that the CRC had missed important socio-cultural and economic realities of the child in Africa (see Table 7.4 for an overview of the ACRWC). To this effect, the Children's Charter addresses African cultural values and experiences, and challenges traditional views, which appear to hinder realization of the rights of the child. The Charter explicitly puts children at the center and argues that children are the centerpiece of society. In effect, the Children's Charter overrules any custom, tradition, cultural or religious practice that fails to reflect the rights, duties, and obligations guaranteed to children under the Charter. The ACRWC defines *a child* as a human being below the age of 18 years. It recognizes the child's unique and privileged place in African society. It also affirms the fact that the African child needs protection and special care. Indeed, as is the case in other parts of the world, children in Africa are at risk for different types of abuse, including economic and sexual exploitation, gender discrimination in education and access to healthcare, as well as involvement in armed conflict (see Table 7.4).

As of May 2013, the ACRWC had been ratified by about 41 of the 54 countries on the continent (African Committee of Experts on the Rights of the Child, n.d.). Zambia, although a signatory to the Charter, has yet to ratify it. In essence, Zambia has expressed its commitment to promote and protect the rights established by the ACRWC, to practice applying these rights, and to interpret the disposition of the ACRWC as required of state parties (African Committee of Experts on the Rights of the Child, n.d.). The country has also, in principle, agreed to submit a report on the status of children to the monitoring body of the ACRWC every three years.

Failure of Zambia to ratify the Charter sends mixed messages. It may be that the children in the country are adequately protected by the legal frameworks in place or that there is little commitment from policy-makers to guarantee safeguards to children. Further, several constraints remain with respect to the ACRWC. These include lack of knowledge of the ACRWC and its mandates. Indeed, the Children's Charter and its activities are largely unknown across the country. This makes accountability problematic. Furthermore, child participation in the public sphere remains mainly on paper. Another point relates to the fact that the Charter

1 Please note that in 2001, the OAU legally became the African Union.

clearly defines government and society as duty-bearers, and children as right-holders, yet Article 31 presents the child as a duty-bearer with responsibilities; introducing confusion in interpretation and harmonization of the Charter into local legal frameworks. And perhaps, the most notable challenge with the Charter is that it devotes little attention to vulnerable children despite the fact that it has been in place for most of the time when vulnerability among children has been on the increase.

Table 7.4 The African Charter on the Rights of a Child

Article	Description/protection guaranteed
1	Defines obligation of state parties
2	Definition of a child
3	Non-discrimination
4	Best interest of the child
5	Survival and development
6	Name and nationality
7	Freedom of expression
8	Freedom of association
9	Freedom of thought, conscience, and religion
10	Protection of privacy
11	Education
12	Leisure, recreation, and cultural activities
13	Handicapped children
14	Health and health services
15	Child labor
16	Protection against child abuse and torture
17	Administration of juvenile justice
18	Protection of the family
19	Parent care protection
20	Parent responsibilities
21	Protection against harmful social and cultural practices
22	Armed conflict
23	Refugee children
24	Adoption
25	Separation from parents
26	Protection against apartheid and discrimination
27	Sexual exploitation
28	Drug abuse
29	Sale, trafficking and abduction
30	Children of imprisoned mothers
31	Responsibility of the child

Source: Created using data from the African Union: http://www.au.int/en/ (p. 149).

The Millennium Development Goals

The United Nations' Millennium Development Goals (MDGs) are one of the most ambitious policy undertakings of the twenty-first century. The MDGs were articulated in 2000 at the United Nations Millennium Summit with eight key areas of focus, including combating poverty, disease, hunger, illiteracy, environmental degradation, and discrimination against women by 2015 (UNDP, 2013; United Nations, 2007, 2010). Generally, MDGs are seen as a global mandate to promote welfare for all, especially the world's vulnerable peoples, so that they can enjoy their basic human rights (UNDP, 2013).

We focus specifically on goals number 2 and 6, which address the rights of children pertaining to: (1) survival; (2) food and nutrition; (3) health and shelter; (4) education; (5) participation; (6) equality; and (7) protection. MGD #2 is concerned with universal primary education. The rationale for this is that the realization of this goal has the potential to enhance progress toward attainment of other Millennium Goals. Moreover, educating children helps reduce poverty and promotes gender equality. In particular, it is inextricably linked to MGD #3—focusing on gender parity in education along with universal primary education. Indeed, universal primary education has been associated with lower child mortality rates and behaviors conducive to the sustainability of the environment (see, e.g., UNICEF, 2004, 2011). Further, school, in the case of OVC, produces many externalities; it offers vulnerable children a safe environment, with support, supervision, and socialization. In school, OVC have an opportunity to learn important life skills with the potential to help them navigate risk. They may also receive life-saving vaccines, fresh water and nutritional supplements. Educating a girl, furthermore, has the potential to dramatically reduce the chance that her offspring will die before the age of five. Moreover, free primary school for all children is a fundamental right to which world governments, including the government of Zambia, committed themselves under the 1989 Convention of the Rights of the Child. As noted, under this goal, the government of Zambia is mandated to facilitate access to primary education and to address issues of gender discrimination and other roadblocks to education, such as user fees and child labor.

Zambia has made headway in the areas of education. The ratio of girls to boys in primary education increased from 0.94 in 2005 to 0.99 by 2010. The observed improvement has been linked to boosts in the infrastructure of primary schools and user friendly policies—e.g., the introduction of policies making free education available to vulnerable children. With regards to secondary education, the ratio of girls to boys declined from 0.92 in 1990 to 0.86 in 2010 (UNDP, 2013). Factors attributed to this include high drop-out rates, lack of income to support school related expenses, and pressure to care for a sick parent (UNDP, 2013).[2] Evaluation of data on tertiary education shows that progress is slow; the ratio of girls to boys is unlikely to be at par by 2015 in Zambia (UNDP, 2013). Indeed, data suggest

2 Evidence suggests girls are likely to drop out of school to care for a sick parent.

that the rate has remained unchanged; it stalled at approximately 0.74 for the period 2003 through 2010 (UNDP, 2013). Although OVC are not the focus of MDG #2, there is existing evidence that the ratio of school attendance of orphans to non-orphans in the 10–14 age group has gone up considerably (Millennium Development Report, 2013; UNDP, 2013). The ratio has increased from 71.8 percent in 2000 to 92 percent in 2009, which is close to the 2015 target of 100 percent (UNDP, 2013).

MGD #6 targets HIV/AIDS and other major diseases such as malaria and tuberculosis. It is well established that the AIDS pandemic affects all sectors of society. For children, the effects are many and complex: ill parents/caregivers are unable to work and support a family; children may be forced to drop out of school to help; orphans may fall prey to violence and even disease including HIV/AIDS (UNICEF, 2010). Under MDG #6, the Zambian government is required to direct effort to several key areas including reducing adolescent risks and vulnerability to HIV/AIDS, increasing access to and use of gender-sensitive sexual and reproductive healthcare, along with making disease-prevention information and skills available.

During the past few years, the Zambian government has organized and conducted information campaigns on HIV/AIDS prevention and treatment. Effort has also been made to increase young people's access to youth-friendly, gender-sensitive health services that provide voluntary testing and counselling, especially in major cities (National AIDS Council, 2012; CSO, 2009). Universal access to treatment for HIV and AIDS and opportunistic disease for children has been put in place. Coupled with this has been an increase in proportion of youth—15–24 years old—with accurate knowledge of HIV and AIDS. In general, the country has made considerable progress towards halting and reversing the spread of HIV and AIDS. Indeed, the number of people infected with HIV has dropped to 14.3 percent of the population. The country has already achieved and surpassed the MDG target for HIV prevalence that was set at 15.6 percent (Millennium Development Report, 2013). These data, although not directly related to OVC, are suggestive—the number of OVC may level off. Despite this progress, HIV incidence (new infections) remains high, especially among young people.

Overall, Zambia has made significant progress in the ratification of international treaties and conventions in connection to the rights of the child. This move has significantly affected the country's response to OVC by ensuring that laws and policies enacted adhere to these global treaties. Overall, the African Charter on the Rights and Welfare of the Child (ACRWC), and Articles 25–29 of the CRC have been the guiding principles for the legal reforms that have been put in place to protect the interests of all children in the country, including OVC.

Other Government Responses: Legal Frameworks that Guide Interventions for OVC at the National Level

Zambia has a comprehensive legal and policy framework to support the country's HIV/AIDS initiatives. Its focus, however, has been primarily on prevention, care, and treatment for adults. This may be explained by the high prevalence rates among adults in the country. During the past few years, however, attention has begun to shift to children, specifically children made vulnerable by the disease (CSO, 2009; National AIDS Council, 2012). The Constitution of the Republic of Zambia, Part III Article #24, establishes provisions for the protection of children. These include protection from child labor, physical and mental exploitation, neglect, and trafficking. Further, two government ministries, the Ministry of Sports, Youth and Child Development (MSYCD) and the Ministry of Community Development and Social Services (MCDSS), are charged with the responsibility of addressing matters related to OVC support (Republic of Zambia, 2010). The MSYCD is largely responsible for legal issues pertaining to the protection of rights while the MCDSS supports delivery of basic social services (Republic of Zambia, 2010). In addition, Zambia has developed a national policy to address concerns of children. In fact, a five-year national strategic plan on OVC has been put in place, under the National Council on AIDS, to enhance coordination at the district and national levels (Republic of Zambia and FNDP, 2006, 2010). Although not directly related to the topic of OVC, a Parliamentary Caucus on Children has been established and endorsed by the Speaker of the National Assembly. As a matter of fact, in 2009 the Parliamentary Caucus Working Group began work on a pilot project to integrate issues related to children into constituency development plans. Further, a National HIV and AIDS Strategic Framework (NASF) has been established with the objective of addressing the needs of people not reached by services and to prevent new infections more effectively (Engle, 2008). Another area of focus has been the provision of welfare through Public Welfare Assistance Schemes (see tables 7.1 and 7.2 for an overview of types of services provided by the government and costs by service domain). In this section we review legal frameworks at the national level. We focus mainly on three: The National Child Policy, Public Welfare Assistance Schemes and the National HIV and AIDS Strategic Framework. We also provide an overview of protection and legal support in relation to vulnerable children.

The National Child Policy

In response to growing vulnerability among children and the need to promote their human development the National Child Policy was put in place in 1994 and revised in 2006 under the patronage of the Ministry of Sports, Youth and Child Development (Republic of Zambia, 2010). Its main objective is to enhance child and youth survival, development and protection through a well-coordinated multi-sector approach. It also aims at strengthening coordination and regulatory framework with regards to the care and protection of children. More specifically it seeks to promote the following principles:

1. rights-based approaches in programming;
2. community participation and empowerment;
3. non-discrimination;
4. gender equality;
5. integrated and holistic service delivery;
6. core cultural values.

The goals and objectives articulated in the National Child Policy were incorporated in the fifth National Development Plan (2006–10). The conceptual framework of the National Child Policy is also reflected in the MDGs. The government has put in place specific targets, strategies, and monitoring plans for achieving them.

Overall, progress has been made in achieving the mandates of the National Child Policy across the country. However, gaps in policy enforcement exist, impeding impact maximization of the National Child Policy on the welfare of OVC. One of the challenges observed is the lack of awareness of the policy in the general public and among the children the policy is designed to protect. Furthermore, lack of monitoring and coordination has been indicated as a problem (Chiwele, 2010; Ministry of Sports, Youth and Child Development, 2012). Indeed, improved coordination would enable organizations at all levels to share experiences of good practice, and facilitate monitoring of resource flows and utilization. In addition, improved monitoring mechanisms would draw attention not only to the needs of OVC but also to the magnitude of the problem and its consequences for the country. Another challenge relates to inadequate funding and leadership. The MSYCD, which is seen as the leader in OVC care, has not played this role effectively due mainly to deficits in funding and personnel (Chiwele, 2010). And perhaps the major point of contention is that the National Child Policy is concerned with the welfare of all children in the country, moving the spotlight from children like OVC who may be experiencing heightened levels of vulnerability.

The National HIV and AIDS Strategic Framework (NASF)

The National HIV and AIDS Strategic Framework was developed in 2006 under the umbrella of the National AIDS Council (NAC) with input from major stakeholders including communities and civil society. Its primary objective is to more effectively prevent new infections and address the needs of people not reached by services (Engle, 2008; UNGASS, 2011). Another objective is to mitigate the socio-economic impacts of HIV and AIDS, especially among the most vulnerable groups, including orphaned and vulnerable children as well as their caregivers. The initiative has, in fact, set the goal of reducing vulnerable households by 50 percent by the year 2015. The NASF facilitates coordination among various ministerial sectors, notably health, education, military, police, women, and youth. In the case of OVC, NASF's mandate is "to protect and provide support." Specifically, it addresses matters pertaining to the provision of basic education, health, and nutrition services, as well as birth registration.

Overall, the NASF has alleviated suffering among vulnerable children in Zambia (Engle, 2008; UNGASS, 2011). The major challenge the scheme faces is lack of funding. Indeed, it is widely documented that funding for OVC and other social services have failed to keep pace with the magnitude of orphans who need care and support (Republic of Zambia, 2010). In fact, available evidence indicates that most of the vulnerable children were still not receiving adequate external support despite implementation of the NASF. For example, the percentage of households with vulnerable children that received basic external aid only increased by about 6 percent between 2005 and 2009. Another problem relates to sustainability—most of the community-based initiatives that have been implemented under the umbrella of the NASF are dependent on external support and hence may not be sustainable in the long run. There is also a marked bias, favoring urban areas in the delivery of services for OVCs (Republic of Zambia, 2010). Further, monitoring and evaluation infrastructure within the country are poorly developed, presenting a challenge to identification of best-practice models. Documentation and information sharing on OVCs intervention and coverage is also poor; as a result there is duplication of programs/services (UNGASS, 2010).

Public Welfare Assistance Schemes (PWAS)

Public Welfare Assistance Schemes are organized under the jurisdiction of the Ministry of Sports, Youth and Child Development (MSYCD) and the Ministry of Community Development and Social Services (MCDSS). These two ministries facilitate coordination and decentralization of national responses to OVC across the country's nine provinces, which are divided in 72 districts. At the head of each scheme is a Provincial Social Welfare Officer who is assisted by District Social Welfare Officers within the province. Each district is further dived into sub-centers run by Community Welfare Assistants and Area Coordinating Committees made up of non-paid volunteers. The District AIDS Task Force (DATF) and the District Welfare Assistance Committee (DWAC), within each province, are responsible for the day-to-day running of the Public Welfare Assistance Schemes (PWAS) (National AIDS Council, 2012).

The primary roles of the PWAS is identification of need and target households, development of collaborations with other community structures for development including Home/Community Health Workers to promote comprehensive outreach, compliance to regulatory guidelines, as well as smooth coordination (National AIDS Council, 2012). Tasks undertaken by the PWAS include the following:

1. implementation of social cash transfer schemes;
2. provision of food security packages/baskets;

3. implementation of women's empowerment initiatives;
4. interpretation of the legal framework for vulnerable people;
5. ensuring cultural sensitive programming;
6. overseeing child protection programs;
7. assisting in disbursement of funds and other support for OVC.

PWAS, for the most part, have been effective in ameliorating hardships for OVC. This is mainly because of their proximity to OVC, permitting effective coordination and decentralization of resources and services. To date, social cash transfer schemes targeting Orphans and Vulnerable Children have been implemented in five rural districts and plans for expansion are underway (Republic of Zambia and UNGASS, 2010). Programs providing food security packages have also been put in place for poor households in six of Zambia's nine provinces. Further, child protection programs are operational in 23 of the country's 72 districts. The challenge remains in the area of funding, dependence on volunteers, limited availability of services in rural localities and sustainability. As noted earlier, externally supported programs are often not sustainable. Further, many of the programs currently in place have been implemented without local input and hence may not effectively respond to local realities.

Legal Protection and Support

As observed, the Ministry of Sport, Youth and Child Development provides legal support and protection to OVC in Zambia. Attention has focused specifically on two areas: birth registration and re-enforcement of inheritance rights for children. Despite this, children continue to struggle against a number of social evils, including property grabbing, a practice in which relatives of the deceased claim the land and other productive assets. Incidences of property grabbing are rampant in the country mainly because customary law, especially in rural localities, does not favor inheritance of property by children. Property grabbing has negative consequences for children. It deprives children of the benefits of intergenerational transfer of wealth, intensifies perceptions of vulnerability and injustice and may heighten strain on the extended family, further weakening its potential to care for vulnerable children. To protect OVC from property grabbing, effort has been put in place to assist parents/caregivers to write wills. Attention has also been directed at ensuring that every child has a birth certificate and national identification (legal documents many children in countries of the global south do not possess), which are necessary in inheritance of property (ACPF, 2008, 2011). Registration of OVC is also essential in ensuring effective delivery of social services.

Overall, progress has been made in the area of legal protection and support. For example, the majority (72 percent) of the children aged 0–5 years in Zambia have had their birth registered. In fact, the data suggests there is no significant difference between OVC and non-OVC in birth registration. Property grabbing, on the other hand, is still an issue of concern despite effort given to writing of wills (Mendenhall et al., 2007; Sloth-Nielsen, 2008). Clearly, a lot needs to be done to ensure children have legal protection. One way to enhance legal protection for vulnerable children is to ensure that legislation reflects the local reality. Alongside this is the need to raise awareness of children's rights to land and other productive assets that are owned by their parents. The fact that child protection, in Zambia, is located within the Ministry of Sport, Youth and Child Development is noteworthy. Indeed, it raises the question of how much attention and resources are channeled to the protection of children.

Responses from Non-Governmental Organizations and Civic Society Institutions

Increases in numbers of OVC, along with the declining capacity of familial networks of care, has prompted a wide range of public groups to assist in the care and support of vulnerable children. These include non-governmental organizations, faith-based organizations, community-based organizations, the private sector, and the business community (tables 7.5 and 7.6 provide an outline of organizations involved with OVC by sector and service domain). There are about 292 non-governmental organizations that have been identified as working with OVC in Zambia. Community- and faith-based organizations make up a significant component of these (see Table 7.5). In this section we focus specifically on three schemes: Strengthening Community Partnership for Empowerment of Orphans and Vulnerable Children (SCOPE-OVC), the Kenneth Kaunda Foundation, and school meals programs.

Table 7.5 Organizations involved with OVC in Zambia by sector (N = 292)

Organization type	Number of organizations
Community-based organizations	138
Faith-based organization	58
Local organizations	53
International organizations	20
Government ministries	10
Statutory bodies	3
Other	10

Source: Created using data from: Center for Global Health & Development Boston University (2010, p. 158).

Table 7.6 Service domains provided to OVC by non-governmental organizations (NGOs)

Service domain	Percentage
Food and nutrition	86
Psychosocial support	76
Education and skill training	67
Child protection	67
Healthcare	57
Shelter and institutional care	48

Note. Service domain categories are not mutually exclusive.
Source: Created using data from Center for Global Health & Development Boston University (2010, p. 158).

Strengthening Community Partnerships for the Empowerment of Orphans and Vulnerable Children

Strengthening Community Partnerships for the Empowerment of Orphans and Vulnerable Children (SCOPE-OVC) is a collaboration of multiple agencies including CARE/Zambia, Family Health International (FHI), United Nation's Children Emergence Fund (UNICEF), and US Agency for International Development (USAID). Other partners are the Ministry of Community Development and Social Services, Ministry of Education, Ministry of Sports, Youth and Child Development as well as faith-based and community-based organizations. The agency focuses on building community capacity with the goal of enabling communities to develop sustainable ways of handling challenges related to OVC. SCOPE-OVC also enables community-based OVC programs to access internal and external support through district and national multi-sector partners. Based on the rationale that keeping children and sibling units together within their extended families and communities may be the best model of OVC care, most of SCOPE-OVC work is at the community and district level.

Areas of focus consist of:

1. education;
2. economic strengthening;
3. food security;
4. psychosocial responses;
5. advocacy;
6. healthcare;
7. capacity building.

Education

SCOPE-OVC has facilitated implementation of community-based schools (defined by the Zambia Community School Secretariat as "community-based, owned, and managed learning institutions") as a grassroots response to the educational needs and aspirations of orphaned and vulnerable children. This has been accomplished mainly through grants offered to community schools. Support from the grants has gone toward the purchase of teaching and learning material, sports equipment, training of community school teachers and peer educators, income-generating activities, and renovation of buildings (SCOPE-OVC, 2009). To date, SCOPE-OVC has given grants to over 42 community schools/groups to benefit OVC.

Economic Strengthening

SCOPE disburses grants to community-based organizations (CBOs) and faith-based organizations (FBOs) to engage in activities aimed at promoting the welfare of OVC. Community-based OVC organizations supported by SCOPE-OVC have been able to carry out group income-generating activities (IGAs). SCOPE-OVC grants have also been given to vulnerable households. Through these grants, SCOPE has facilitated microfinance training programs, acquisition of skills in managing small businesses, management of revolving loan funds, as well as linkages to microcredit. As a result of this effort, vulnerable households are able to access credit, manage businesses, and provide for the needs of OVC in their care. Economic strengthening has also involved attempts to address food security through agricultural inputs and food baskets. Households have been trained and supported in the use of appropriate technologies and farming methods (SCOPE-OVC, 2009).

Psychosocial Responses

Recognizing that responding to psychosocial needs may be a critical but mostly ignored part in the care of orphans and children with a parent living with HIV/AIDS, SCOPE-OVC has supported community-led activities aimed at building the capacity of communities to cope and better deal with issues of loss and grief. More specifically, SCOPE-OVC has provided support through psychosocial experts who have developed training materials for community members as well as guidelines outlining social practices to better meet the emotional needs of children. Psychosocial support also includes the training of community caregivers. In addition, SCOPE-OVC has supported the establishment of community-based camps to provide respite to vulnerable children.

Advocacy

Working through and with district and national partners from multiple sectors, SCOPE-OVC has enabled advocacy for the rights of OVC. Advocacy efforts have involved challenges around normal child development, nurturing, HIV/AIDS infection, and affection along with awareness and prevention. Advocacy initiatives have heightened stakeholder understanding of the situation of OVC, introducing an informed perspective on decisions regarding OVC programming. It has also underscored the role of human rights in the welfare of the child considered vulnerable.

Capacity Building

In the districts where it is present, SCOPE-OVC has developed and strengthened the capacity of district and community-level OVC organizations with the goal of enabling them to better address the situation of orphaned and vulnerable children. Capacity building, from SCOPE-OVC's point of view, is closely connected to the needs of districts and communities. This perspective has enabled SCOPE-OVC to assist with prioritizing unique community and household needs and identifying local resources to meet detected needs. Capacity building has taken different forms and covers financial management, organizational skills, fund raising, proposal writing, and various OVC technical interventions, such as psychosocial support and skill building. Another important area that SCOPE-OVC has been involved in, with respect to capacity building, is improvement of monitoring and evaluation. The network has established monitoring and evaluation frameworks in four districts including Lusaka, Livingstone, Kitwe, and Mongu (SCOPE-OVC, 2009). The data collected has been instrumental in the development of responsive community-led interventions.

In general, SCOPE work with community and district partners has been effective. To date, the scheme has been implemented in 12 districts across the country and has reached over 137,521 orphans and vulnerable children with life-sustaining care and support services (UNICEF, 2008). Moreover, there is general consensus that strengthening community capacity may be the only viable way for building effective, sustainable support systems for children experiencing vulnerability (see, e.g., Kawilila, 2006; Richter et al., 2009; UNICEF, 2011). The effort to strengthen communities and district capacity has improved coordination and reduced overlap in OVC programming service delivery. The program has also enhanced community cohesion. The major challenge with respect to SCOPE-OVC is its heavy reliance on external funding and lack of meaningful participation by primary stakeholders.

School Meals: World Food Program (WFP)

Provision of school meals as an intervention for OVC started in 2003 in the aftermath of the food and drought crisis of 2002. The initiative was implemented with support from the UN's World Food Programme (WFP) in partnership with Project Concern International (PCI). The initiative targets community-based schools and centers that cater to street children. The primary objectives of the program are:

1. to improve school enrolment and attendance;
2. to increase the participation of HIV/AIDS affected households in activities with potential to improve their health and livelihood;
3. to improve HIV/AIDS-related knowledge and practices in the target population;
4. to improve the capacity of implementing partners to execute and manage the program.

The program provides one cooked meal per day to participating school children. This consists of a wet ration of High Energy Protein Supplement (HEPS) and a locally produced fortified soy blend donated by WFP and delivered by PCI. The food rations are prepared on-site by school volunteers. All children in the target community schools are provided the ration to avoid stigma. In addition to the school meal, children identified as particularly vulnerable receive a monthly family take-home ration consisting of a 50 kilogram bag of grain. This targeting takes into account the economic and social status of homes with child-headed households—households considered particularly vulnerable. Community School Coordinators have been trained in the various aspects of managing school-based feeding programs including community mobilization strategies, food preparation and handling, as well as basic hygiene. Another component of this program is Behavior Change Communication (BCC) providing information on HIV/AIDS through drama, song, and dance.

So far, school feeding programs have served over 205 community schools, as well as nine residential centers in the country. Overall, enrollment and attendance rates have improved considerably in participating schools. Despite this, challenges exist. The large number of children attending community-based schools may represent children excluded from the formal school system. Monitoring of program effect, sustainability, and the question of dependence still remain largely unexplored. The question of "foreign hand syndrome" stands as another challenge.

The Kenneth Kaunda Children of Africa Foundation (KKCAF)

This is seen an example of a community-based approach to alleviate the needs of children experiencing vulnerability. In response to the enormity of needs presented by OVC, the foundation has established day care centers, commonly referred to as children's villages, in five high-density locations of Lusaka to provide respite and care as well as meals, education, and medical attention to children while they continue to live in their own homes. Children served range in age from about three to nine years. People from the community, for the most part, assume the responsibility of the day-to-day running of the day care centers. Adults from the community, through visits and supervision, ensure that the living conditions of children living alone are reasonable. In fact, subjective evidence indicates that some communities, by consensus, have appointed designated caregivers to monitor and support children who live on their own.

The centers have served numerous OVC in the city of Lusaka. They also offer services to people living with HIV/AIDS. Data on the effects of the children's centers on OVC served, to our knowledge, is currently not available. The model is a fairly recent undertaking. Anecdotal evidence is that the scheme is a viable way of addressing the needs of OVC because it is community-based and, hence, reflects the needs of OVC better. Challenges with this approach to care include lack of a formalized regulatory or monitoring mechanism as well as standards for the living arrangements of children in child-headed households.

Conclusion

Zambia's commitment to the survival, wellbeing, and development of children in a safe environment is articulated in ratification of international treaties and national policies, plans, and programs. Overall, headway has been made in enhancing the welfare of OVC through implementation of progressive policies that are guided by major international instruments that the government of Zambia has ratified. Despite the noted gains, obstacles to effective HIV prevention, treatment, care and support for vulnerable groups, notably children, continue to exist.

At the policy level, although parliament has ratified laws that increased penalties for the sexual abuse of children, and provided firmer regulation concerning the participation of children in paid employment, currently, there is no legislation that overtly bans discrimination and stigmatization of persons affected and/or infected by HIV (UNGASS, 2010). Furthermore, lack of well-defined legal and regulatory protection for OVC continues to be a problem. For example, guidelines provided under customary laws tend to be contradictory with respect to inheritance and ownership of property by women and children (UNGASS, 2010, 2011). This makes inheritance of property by OVC problematic. Another area of concern relates to the definition of the child. The country has multiple age thresholds that are used to define a child. For instance, customary law defines a child as anyone below the age of 14 years, while the Marriage Act sets the age of 21 years as the age of sexual consent, and the constitution of the Republic of Zambia offers multiple definitions (Republic of Zambia, 1996). The lack of a standard with respect to how to define a child in Zambia may be problematic in that it may encourage misinterpretation of the law, placing children at a disadvantage. Coupled with the above is the lack or limited participation of children in decision-making. Despite initiatives like the Youth Parliament, it is well established that formal and informal initiatives responding to vulnerable children have been implemented with little involvement of children and their communities (Germann et al., 2008; Tiaji, 2005; UNESCO, 2010). As a result, decision and programs continue to be undertaken without the input of the primary stakeholders. In addition, there is some evidence to suggest that assistance to OVC continues to be hampered by inadequate funding and a lack of coordination among schemes charged with the responsibility of OVC care (UNGASS, 2010).

Another challenge relates to the fact that children in Zambia are generally not aware of their rights nor the means of redress available to them and hence do not make a claim (ACPF, 2011; African Committee of Experts on the Rights of the Child, n.d.). This is especially the case in rural areas. Indeed, the few children that may be aware of their rights nationwide are often privileged and have their needs adequately addressed, and therefore are less likely to have their rights violated. The situation for a typical Zambian child, especially OVC, who has been denied her rights is lamentable; the child is likely to experience maltreatment, abuse, and neglect, inhibiting her life chances and opportunity to dream and aspire for tomorrow (Chishimba and Kaela, 2006; UNICEF, 2010). Also, policies targeting vulnerable children are just being created despite the fact that vulnerability among children has been on the increase since the early 1990s.

With respect to programming, while great strides have been made in implementation of community-based initiatives that support OVC, the focus has been primarily on the provision of basic needs and psychosocial support at the expense of other unique needs that characterize vulnerable children (SAFAIDS, 2012). Indeed, existing evidence suggest that 86 percent of services targeted at OVC fall in the area of food and nutrition (OVC-CARE Project, 2009). While this is important, it does not take into account other critical needs such as information on life-skills, socio-cultural skills, awareness of rights, and other skills that OVC might need in navigating their world and making informed decisions (SAFAIDS, 2012). Moreover, limitations in outreach to OVC still persist. Only about 10 percent of OVC have access to care and support outside of the familial network. Mechanisms for research and evaluation are also weakly developed. As has been observed by others, poor documentation and sharing of information on OVC intervention makes replication of best practices difficult (UNGASS, 2010, 2011). It also means that programming decisions continue to be loosely guided by evidence from the field.

Finally, it is general knowledge that OVC programming is dependent on external funding. Indeed, donor support has and continues to provide life-sustaining services to OVC. This is laudable. However, it may obscure the chain of accountability that exists between a government and the people it is mandated to serve. Governments, even in poor countries of sub-Saharan Africa, have the moral responsibility and authority to respond to the challenge presented by OVC.

The primary role of government, in this regard, is not advocacy—calling on the international community to act—but to develop sustainable solutions. In the long run, the country will bear the cost of failing children in terms of squandered potential, loss of productivity, and loss of political voice. Indeed, vulnerability among children has the potential to weaken the very social fabric that holds families, communities, and the country together.

Bibliography

African Child Policy Forum (ACPF) (2008). In the Best Interests of the Child: Harmonising Laws on Children in Eastern and Southern Africa. http://www.africanchildinfo.net.

African Child Policy Forum (ACPF) (2011). In the Best Interests of the Child: Harmonising Laws on Children in West and Central Africa. http://www.africanchildinfo.net.

African Committee of Experts on the Rights of the Child (ACERWC) (n.d.). Launch of the ACERWC general comments. http://acerwc.org/523/.

African Committee of Experts on the Rights and Welfare of the Child, African Union, The. http://www.africa-union.org/child/home.htm.

Africa's Orphaned and Vulnerable Generations: Children Affected by AIDS (2006). New York: UNICEF/UNAIDS.

Besley, M.A. (2005). *AIDS and the Family: Policy Options for a Crisis in Family Capital*. New York: United Nations.

Center for Global Health & Development Boston University (2010). OVC-CARE project: The scale, scope and impact of alternative care for OVC in developing countries. Boston, MA. http://www.bu.edu/cghd/files/2009/12/The-Scale-Scope-and-Impact-of-Alternative-Care-for-OVC-Full-Report-2.12.10.pdf.

Central Statistical Office (CSO) (2009). *Zambia Demographic and Health Survey 2007*. Calverton: ORC-Macro, with Central Statistics Office, Lusaka.

Chatterji, M., Hutchinson, P., Murray, N., et al. (2010). *Evaluating the Impact of Community-based Interventions on Schooling Outcomes among Orphans and Vulnerable Children in Lusaka, Zambia*. Vulnerable Children and Youth Studies.

Chishimba, S. and Kaela, G. (2006). A Glimpse into the African Child's Future in an Era of HIV/AIDS: The Case for Zambia. Presented at the International Conference on AIDS. http://www.aegis.com/conferences/iac/2006/MoPE0253.pdf.

Chiwele, D.K. (2010). *Assessing Administrative Capacity and Costs of Cash Transfer Schemes in Zambia*. International Policy Centre for Inclusive Growth, Country Study, February 2010.

Devereux, S. and Wood, D. (2008). Zambia's Social Cash Transfer Pilot Schemes: A Review Report for the Technical Working Group on Social Assistance, September 2008.

Dunn, A. and Parry-Williams, J. (2008). *Alternative Care for Children in Southern Africa: Progress, Challenges and Future Directions*. Nairobi: UNICEF, Social Policy and Social Protection Cluster.

Engle, P. (2008). National Plans of Action for Orphans and Vulnerable Children in sub-Saharan Africa: Where are the youngest children? Working Paper No. 50. The Hague, the Netherlands: Bernard van Leer Foundation.

Germann, S., Wamimbi, R., and Ngoma, F. (2008). CRC Article 12 and 13—Right of Participation and Freedom of Expression. A Study on Child Participation and Freedom of Expression in Community Owned Coordination Approaches to Provide Care and Support to Children made Vulnerable by HIV and AIDS. Presented at the AIDS 2008—XVII International AIDS Conference.

Government of the Republic of Zambia, Living Conditions Monitoring Survey Report 2006 and 2010 (2011). Lusaka: Central Statistical Office.

Government of the Republic of Zambia, First Draft Constitution of the Republic of Zambia (2012). Lusaka: Technical Committee on Drafting the Zambian Constitution.

Health and Development and Health and Development Africa (2010). USAID/ Project SEARCH, September 10, 2010.

Hutchinson, P. and Thurman, T. (2009). *Analyzing the Cost Effectiveness of Interventions to Benefit OVC: Evidence from Kenya and Tanzania, USAID*, Measure Evaluation.

Kawilila, S. (2006). It Takes a Village to Raise a Child: Community Response to HIV/AIDS and Plight of Orphan. Presented at the AIDS 2006—XVI International AIDS Conference. http://aids2006.org/Abstracts/A2193108.aspx.

Kirkpatrick, S., Rojjanasrirat, W., South, B., et al. (2012). Assessment of Emotional Status of Orphans and Vulnerable Children in Zambia. *Journal of Nursing Scholarship*, 44(2), 194–201.

Living Condition Monitoring Survey (2006). Republic of Zambia Central Statistics Office. http://www.unicef.org/har09/files/har09_Zambia_countrychapter.pdf.

Malcom, C. (2009). Happy Shopper? The problem with service user and carer participation. *British Journal of Social Work*, 39, 179–88.

Millennium Development Report (MDR) (2013). *Assessing progress in Africa towards the Millennium Development Goals*. Washington, DC.

Mendenhall, E. et al. (2007). Property grabbing and will writing in Lusaka, Zambia: An examination of wills of HIV infected cohabiting couples. *AIDS Care*, 19(3), 369–374.

Ministry of Education Census (2009). MoE, Zambia Annual School Census (Lusaka 2010); MoE, A Review of the Re-entry Policy.

Ministry of Sports, Youth and Child Development (MSYCD) (2012). *Orphaned and Vulnerable Children in Zambia*. Zambia 2004 Situation Analysis.

Mugabe, M., Stirling, M., and Whiteside, A. (2002). *Future Imperfect: Protecting Children on the Brink*. Presented at the African Leadership Consultant: Urgent Action for Children on the brink. Johannesburg, 9–10 September.

National AIDS Council (2012). *Zambia Country Report: Monitoring the Declaration of Commitment on HIV and AIDS and the Universal Access* (biennial report). Republic of Zambia: Author.

Nkhoma, S., Khan, N., Chipanta, D., and Bhatt, P. (2008). Responding to OVC in Zambia through the Lens of the National Child Policy. Presented at the AIDS 2006—XVI International AIDS Conference. http://aids2008.org/Abstracts/A2192919.aspx.

OVC-CARE Project (2009). *Zambia Research Situation Analysis on Orphans and Other Vulnerable Children*. Boston University Center for Global Health and Development.

Republic of Zambia (amended 1996). The Constitution. http://www.wipo.int/wipolex/en/details.jsp?id=5394.

Republic of Zambia Ministry of Finance and National Planning (2009). Mid-Term Review of the Fifth National Development Plan.

Richter, L. (2004). The Impact of HIV/AIDS on the Development of Children [monograph]. *A Generation at Risk? HIV/AIDS, Vulnerable Children and Security in Southern Africa*, 109, 9–31.

Richter, L.M., Sherr, L., Adato, M., et al. (2009). Strengthening Families to Support Children Affected by HIV and AIDS. *AIDS Care*, 21(S1), 3–12.

SAFAIDS (2012). Discussion summary: Engaging traditional leaders in HIV and GBV prevention. http://catalogue.safaids.net/publications/discussion-summary-engaging-traditional-leaders-hiv-and-gbv-prevention.

SCOPE-OVC (2009). Family Health International/Zambia, SCOPE-OVC: Final Project Review Report.

Skinner, D., Tsheko, N., Mtero-Munyati, S., et al. (2006). Towards a Definition of Orphaned and Vulnerable Children. *AIDS Behavior*, 10, 619–26.

Sloth-Nielsen, J. (2008). A Developing Dialogue—Child Rights, Children's Law and Economics: Surveying Experiences from Southern and Eastern African Law Reform Processes. *Electronic Journal of Comparative Law*, 12(3).

Tiaji, S.B. (2005). IDS orphans and vulnerable children (OVC): Problems, responses, and issues for Congress. Congressional Research Service. http://www.sarpn.org/documents/d0001829/index.php.

UNDP (2013). Human Development Report—Zambia. http://hdr.undp.org/en/countries/profiles/ZMB.

UNDP (2013). Human Development Index 2013. http://hdr.undp.org/en/media/HDR2013_EN_Summary.pdf.

UNDP (2013). *Millennium Development Goals: Progress Report—Zambia*. Zambia: UNDP.

UNESCO (2010). *EFA Global Monitoring Report. Reaching the Marginalized.* Paris.

UNGASS (2010). Zambia Country Progress Report. http://data.unaids.org/pub/Report/2010/zambia_2010_country_progress_report_en.pdf.

UNGASS (2011). *Zambia Country Progress Report: Monitoring the Declaration of Commitment on HIV and AIDS and the Universal Access*. Submitted to the United Nations General Assembly Special Session on HIV and AIDS.

UNICEF (2004). The Framework for the Protection, Care and Support of Orphans and Vulnerable Children Living in a World with HIV and AIDS. *Technical and Policy Documents, UNICEF*. http://www.unicef.org/aids/files/Framework_English.pdf.

UNICEF (2005). *Every Child's Birth Right. Inequalities and Trends in Birth Registration*. New York: UNICEF.

UNICEF (2008). *Zambia: Situational Analysis of Children and Women 2008*. Zambia: UNICEF.

UNICEF (2010). *Progress for Children: Achieving the MDGs with Equity*. Number 9, September. New York.

UNICEF (2011). Taking Evidence to Impact: Making a Difference for Vulnerable Children Living in a World with HIV and AIDS, 1–78. http://www.unicef.org/eapro/TAKING_EVIDENCE_TO_IMPACT_FINAL.pdf.

UNICEF (2013). The State of the World's Children 2013. http://www.unicef.org/sowc2013/.

United Nations (2007). United National General Assembly Political Declaration on HIV/AIDS. 2006. 60/262.

United Nations (2010). World Population Prospects: The 2010 Revision.

Wallis A., Dukay V., and Mellins C. (2010). Power and empowerment: Fostering effective collaboration in meeting the needs of orphans and vulnerable children. *Global Public Health*, 5(5), 509–522.

Zambia Demographic Health Survey (ZDHS) (2013–14). https://dhsprogram.com/pubs/pdf/FR304/FR304.pdf.

Zambia Human Development Report (ZDHR) (2007). Zambia country report: Monitoring the declaration of commitment on HIV and AIDS and the universal access. http://www.unaids.org/sites/default/files/country/documents/ZMB_narrative_report_2014.pdf.

Zambia National Response to HIV/AIDS Project: CRAIDS Annual Report (2006). Lusaka: Ministry of Finance and National Planning.

PART IV
The Voices of the Children

Chapter 8
Children Speak Out: Is Anyone Listening?

Margaret Lombe and Alex Ochumbo

Overview of the Chapter

This chapter supplements the literature reviewed with evidence from research conducted from children in Zambia and Kenya. Data were collected from children in institutional care as well as child-headed households (N = 178). Our goal was to fully capture the children's perception of their situation and experiences; hence, the data is mainly descriptive.

Description of the Data

As noted, data were collected from children in institutional care in Kenya (N = 88) and in child-headed households in Zambia (N = 90). The questionnaire covered a wide range of issues, these are reviewed below.

- Demographics: This included age, gender, place of residence, school enrollment and grade level.
- Respondent and HIV/AIDS: This question addressed issues around a respondents' knowledge, perception, status, and acquaintance with HIV/AIDS.
- Respondent's Family (Relationship with family members): This question looked at whether/or not a respondent's parents are dead, cause of death, age at parent's death, feeling about parents' death and reasons for feeling that way.
- Relationship with Relatives (Relationship with community): The focus is on whether or not a respondents is visited by relatives, feelings when visited or not visited, reaction to the visit, what relatives say, how they relate, explanation of relationship, what they want to hear from relatives, why they want to hear this, what they would like their relatives to do for them and why.
- Respondent's Education (Experiences with the home/institutions): This addressed a respondent's reasons for going to school and whether or not school is important to them and why.

- Respondent's Goals and Future: The question asked respondents to list their goals, assistance to attain the goals, what they felt children classified as OVC needed to attain their goals.
- Human Rights (The rights of the child as defined in the Convention on the Rights of the Child): The focus was on whether or not the respondent has heard of human rights, what they mean, whether children should have rights, whether these should be the same as adult's rights, view on children's rights, which ones are important and whether respondents enjoyed them. In addition, an explanation of rights attained, who is responsible for making them be realized, and what would be done to ensure children's rights were known and respected, was required.
- Life at the Home/Institution (Experiences with the home/institutions): This question asked about life at home or institution, whether the child/children were happy at the institution/home and why, length of time of residence at the institution/home, and things that could be done to improve the lives of children in these locations.
- Their voices on how vulnerable children should be treated: This question focused on treatment of children classified as OVC by other children and adults and reasons for the perceived treatment. It also addressed the issue of how these children would like to be treated by others.

Part A: Experiences of Child-Headed Households in Zambia: Observations from the Field

Experiences of children in child-headed households vary. They are determined by a number of factors including finances, strength of familial ties and community cohesion to mention a few. Communities and other systems of care focus on provision of basic needs and short-term care for children in child-headed households, e.g., food, clothing, shelter and to some extent healthcare, and education. Little attention is focused on meeting their emotional needs, nurturing and the need for security. In this section we draw upon data from the study we conducted to capture the perception of affected children. The survey in question was conducted in Zambia's copper-belt province, and targeted children in child-headed households (N = 90). The survey asked the children questions related to their status as well as experiences (for examples of the questions refer to Appendix A). A summary of the content of the questionnaire is given in the data description section that follows.

Background

In recent years, there has been a noted increase in the number of children living alone, in what have come to be known as child-headed households (Care Kenya, 2004; Foster and Williamson, 2000). These children often assume adult responsibilities when they are still relatively young. Child-headed households emerged because surviving relatives are not able to absorb the orphans into their households. The extended family may have reached its absorptive capacity. Child-headed households represent one extreme on the continuum of the pragmatic ways of providing for children rendered vulnerable by the epidemic and other factors. Children in such households are the focus of this section.

Demographic characteristics of the sub-sample

The age of the children in the study sample ranged from 13 to 20 years with an average age of 15–17 (71.0 percent). By gender, 72 percent of the children were male. All the children were currently enrolled in school, and about 95 percent of the children were in secondary school. Most of the respondents (62.8 percent) indicated that they were between the ages of 1 and 14 when they lost a parent/s. All the respondents currently live in a child-headed household.

Children and HIV/AIDS

Most of the children in the study sample have heard of HIV/AIDS and their perception of it is that Acquired Immune Deficiency Syndrome is a drastic virus. The children believe AIDS is an incurable, killer disease caused by a virus which kills red blood cells that protect the body. It attacks the immune system of the body. It is real and has taken the lives of many people. The children reported the virus is transmitted through various ways such as sexual intercourse, using unsterilized needles or blades. All the respondents from Zambia were not infected but knew of someone—a sister, cousin, aunt, brother, uncle or neighbor, and friend—who was HIV positive.

Children and the family (relationship with family members)

With respect to their perception about their parents—whether dead or alive, and cause of death, some of the children indicated that they had lost their parents through HIV/AIDS when they were very young. Others do not know the cause of their parents' death, while some of the children reported that their parents died of: diabetes, HIV, TB, malaria, stomach problems, high blood pressure, and road accident. The majority of the children (70 percent) said that they were sad, unhappy, lonely, insecure and miserable, in pain, and even worried when they think about the death of their parents. Some feel like taking their own lives—"it is as if the world is over," they said. Others indicated being at peace—they feel God takes care of them. Reasons for the reported feelings included:

- inability to afford school fees and food;
- challenges of growing up without parental care;
- hearing friends talk about their own parents who are still alive when they never had a chance to see theirs;
- living in abject poverty;
- loneliness;
- missing their parents.

Another aspect of familial connection is visits from relatives. A significant number of children (74.4 percent) indicated that they received visits/care from relatives. When visited by relatives these children say that they feel loved, appreciated, noble, satisfied, excited and less worried. Overall, children who did not get visits from their relatives did not dwell on their feelings. Many of them noted that this could be for various reasons, including time commitment, lack of resources and relatives living in other parts of the country.

It is important to note that during the visits, the children would like to hear certain things said by their relatives. They would like to be encouraged about education and told to work hard; to be told that they are remembered and accepted; that they are loved and will continue to be cared for. They also felt that relatives need to talk about the children's deceased parents. Comforting them by telling them that the future will be bright for them despite their loss, is another expression of support that the children value. Some children reported that they would like to receive their relatives; to them this is an important sign of acceptance and appreciation.

The children in the study sample also indicated that they see education as important for their future; it is the key to success. They also feel that it is important for them to be appreciated; it makes them happy. According to the children, relatives are a gift from God and their encouragement has the potential to impact the children's lives positively. The children also reported that they would like to make their relatives proud of them. They see this as materializing with their success. Perhaps, one of the important observations emerging from this discussion was the children's need for support and encouragement with school related matters—grades, payment of school fees, and provision of a stable home environment for them.

Children and education

Almost all the children (95.3 percent) in the study sample indicated that they were happy to go to school. They saw this as being "cool." They also indicated that education was the key to a better life—the life they aspired for. With education, the children pointed out, they would be able to take care of themselves and their relatives. All the children agreed that education is important because it leads to development of the individual and has a positive impact on national development. Some of the children saw education as a vehicle to wealth—these indicated that they would like to be rich when they complete their education.

Children and goals for the future

Most of the children in the study sample reported positive goals for the future. These were exemplified mainly in career options such as: Journalism, medicine, accountancy, teaching, law and nursing. Most of the respondents aspired to a life free of poverty and said they wanted to be "someone" in life. To attain these goals, 95 percent of them indicated that they depended on the support of grandparents and other relatives.

Children speak about human rights

A significant number of children (93 percent) indicated that they had heard of human rights. The children in the study sample all believe that children should have rights. A considerable number (74.4 percent) of them, however, do not believe that children should have the same rights as adults.

The following is what human rights mean to these children:

- a right is a lawful claim or benefit you expect from the community;
- this is the freedom a citizen gains from the people around them, including the community;
- freedom to do what one wants;
- freedom that a human being has to do something; it is a condition that allows people to live freely;
- it means to know one's rights;
- it means every human being has a right to life;
- it is the benefit you expect from community, government and parents;
- this is the authority people are given for them to live a full life;
- they are conditions of life that allows the person to live freely.

Children's views of the rights of the child

Children feel that adults have the rights to do what they like but children should have rights as well "because we are all human beings." They felt that adults are much older than children, they know more and can do difficult things that children cannot do so they should have more rights and responsibilities. About 23.2 percent of the respondents had the view that children are different from adults and should have their own rights—have rights according to their level. These included the right to education, food and shelter as well as parental care among many others. Rights seen as important by children in the study sample are presented in Figure 8.1.

A significant proportion of children (93 percent) reported that, despite their OVC status, they enjoyed many of the rights mentioned. With respect to why the mentioned rights should be attained, they argued that the right to education, for example, will enable them have a better future. They also felt that rights made them feel protected. They pointed out that rights gave them the freedom of expression to speak their mind. Slightly more than half of children in the study sample (55.8 percent) see others, including teachers, institutions (e.g., schools) and community, as responsible for helping them realize their rights. To ensure that rights are attained the children said that they would use institutions such as schools and teachers, parents, the community. They felt teachers should be key in helping them both know and realize their rights.

Regarding respecting children's rights, the children felt, generally, that their rights were not respected. They felt that organizations, especially schools, could help ensure that their rights were respected. They also felt that anyone who failed to respect children and their rights should be reported to the police, and be

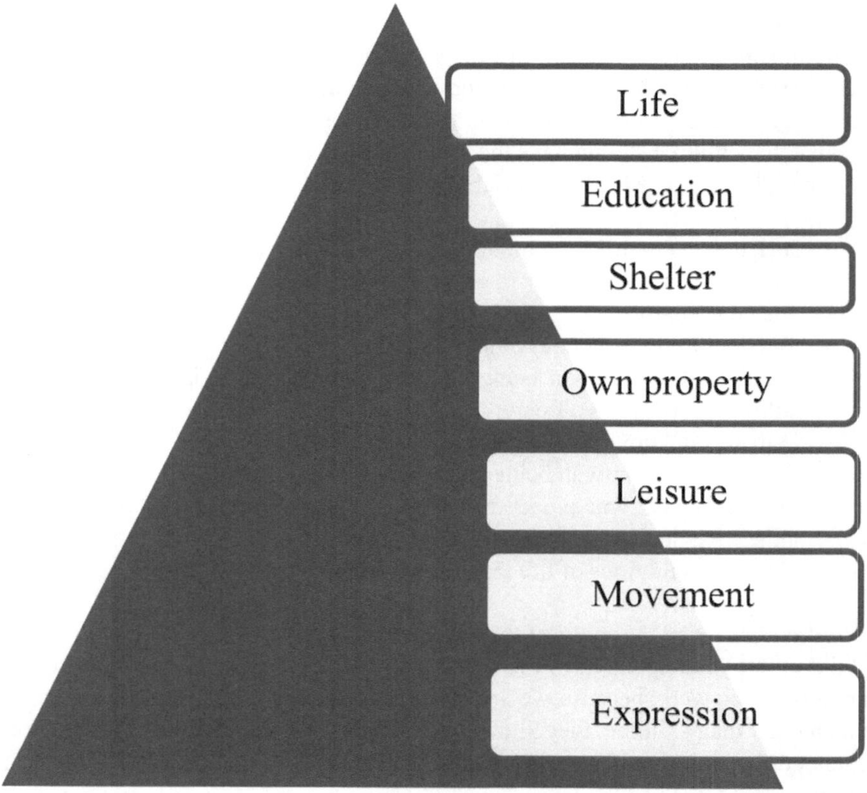

Figure 8.1 Rights rated as important
Source: Authors' own data.

prosecuted or punished. They indicated the need for periodic inquiry from children with respect to whether or not their rights were respected. They pointed out that this role could be played by the government.

Experiences of children in child-headed households
About half (46.6 percent) of the children interviewed reported that they were happy at home. This was mainly because the children were able to live together as a family unit. Others, however, indicated that life was hard and challenging. Reasons given for this are organized below (see Figure 8.2).

Most of the children said that they would make the following changes to improve the lives of children classified as vulnerable:

- encourage them to go to school and study hard;
- build community schools or come up with community organizations to help children;

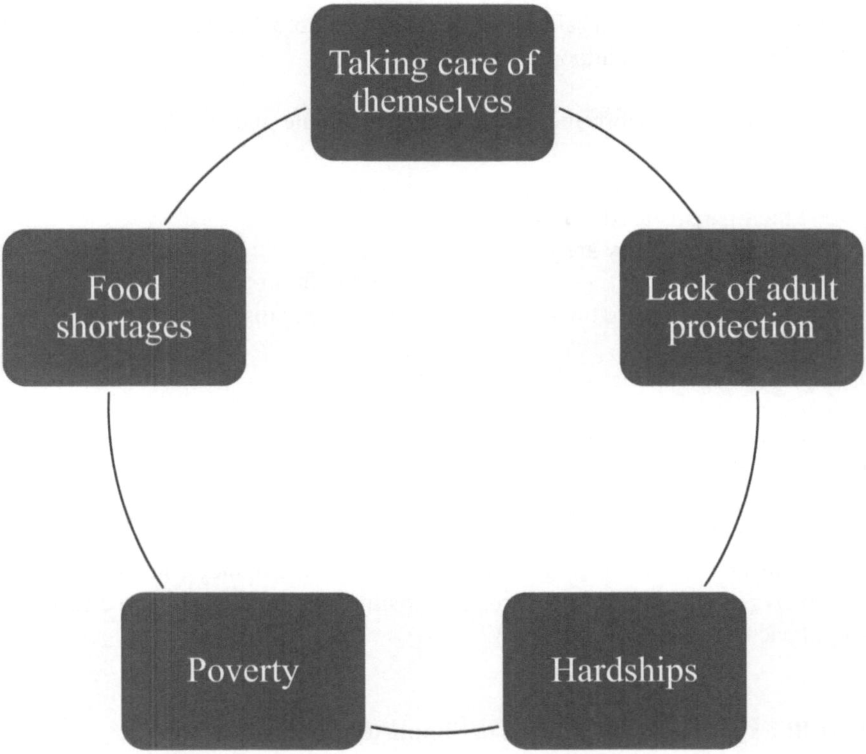

Figure 8.2 Challenges experienced by children in child-headed households
Source: Authors' own data.

- constructing new schools and new hostels so children can complete their education and get good jobs;
- improve health and care;
- create school funds;
- provide them with food and clothing.

Children's voices on treatment of vulnerable children
Most of the children (60.5 percent) reported being well/fairly treated by their peers. The children gave the following reasons for the way they are treated by others:

- their friends know them well;
- their friends/peers love them;
- they are good friends, others should treat them the same way;
- they respect others—do unto others what you would like them to do to you;
- they are sharp and accurate at school and do not hurt others;
- they are seen as deserving of help/acceptance.

All the children surveyed said that they would like to be treated fairly and not be pitied. They feel this is important because:

- they need support, they are responsible people and should not be treated like babies;
- they are human beings and their rights have to be respected;
- their parents used to treat them well;
- it shows that they are loved and respected;
- even in difficult times, they can think of the future;
- it is important for their development into good citizens.

What the children in the study sample would do to help other orphans and vulnerable children

The majority (75 percent) of respondents indicated that they would invest in helping children classified as OVC. Investment indicated ranged from provision of education, sponsorship, provision of shelter, food, clothes, medicines and good healthcare. Other supports reported include building orphanages, building places of worship and recreation, and making money available so they could have a good life. With regards to OVC who are HIV positive the children observed that they would encourage them to take ARVs.

Part B: Experiences of Children in Supported Facilities in Kenya: Observations from the Field

Nyumbani Children's Home

Background

The home was founded to provide holistic care for HIV-positive children, who are mostly orphans. It is part of the Children of God Relief Institute (COGRI). The home takes on the structure of a small village/community and is organized in family units. Children are placed in a family unit headed by a house parent—father/mother. At a later stage, the young people are moved to a Youth Centre in preparation for their re-insertion into the wider community. While at the home, the children receive life skills training through organized seminars and peer counseling. Data utilized in this section were collected from children at the home (N = 47).

Demographic characteristics of the sub-sample

The children were aged between 12 and 20 years, with the majority being between the ages of 14 to 16 (55.3 percent). With respect to gender, 51.1 percent of the children were male. Nearly all the respondents are currently attending school (97.9 percent). In fact, most of them are in upper primary and lower secondary school (80.8 percent). Most of the respondents in this sub-sample have lost a parent/s

(93.6 percent). About half of the children (53.2 percent) reported being between the ages of one and nine when their parent/s died. All the respondents resided at Nyumbani Children's Home in Nairobi, Kenya. About half of the children (46.8 percent) have lived at the home between 1 and 16 years.

Children and HIV/AIDS: Knowledge, perception, status and acquaintance with AIDS

The children's perceptions of HIV/AIDS did not vary greatly. For the majority, AIDS is a deadly disease caused by the HIV virus and has no cure. Others saw it as a killer disease which is not as bad as cancer but infectious in many ways. A few respondents see AIDS as a harmful virus which is caused by blood transfusion, passed from mother to child, and careless behavior.

With regards to their HIV status, 46.8 percent of the children reported that they were not infected by the HIV virus while 51.1 percent of them indicated that they were HIV positive. About half of the respondents (48.9 percent) indicated that that they knew someone who has AIDS. The relationship between the child and HIV/AIDs infected person ranged from friend to close relative.

Children and the family (relationship with family members)

The majority of the children were less than five years old when their parents died, and so have little recollection of their parents. These children have little knowledge of what caused the death of their parent/s. For the few who remember they reported that their parent/s died of HIV/AIDS, cancer and other diseases. It is important to note that close to half of the children did not respond to this question.

In terms of the children's feelings about the death of their parents, these varied a great deal and were determined by whether or not the child had a recollection of her parent/s and her assessment of her current situation. A considerable proportion of the children (36 percent) had trouble answering this question because they never knew their parents. Others (27 percent) feel that something "big" is missing from their lives. Some (about 9 percent) reported being angry when they think about their parents. Yet others (about 21 percent) reported feeling sad and lonely because they did not have the family love that parents provide. A small number of children (6.3 percent) did not want to talk about their parents. A number of the children indicated that they feel rejected and that God was unfair to them when they think of their parents.

When asked why they felt that way, their responses were as follows:

- they never saw their parents;
- God gives and takes;
- the special bond between children and parents was missing;
- did not have the chance to interact and know their parents;
- do not get the support they need;
- they are not taken good care of or effectively nurtured;
- they just do not know what to feel;

- life without one's parents is tough;
- seeing other children with their parents;
- missing them even though their image is not clear;
- it brings a lot of pain and sorrow.

With regards to the children's relationship with their relatives, the majority of children reported visits from the extended family (70.2 percent). Their feeling about the extended family varied considerably. A significant proportion of the children (53 percent) said that they enjoyed visits from the extended family. They added that this made them feel appreciated and hopeful about the future. It made them feel that people care about them and love them. It showed that they belong, have roots somewhere, and a family outside of the institution. The children look at their relatives with appreciation and thank God for them. The children who had little or no contact with the extended family reported feelings of sadness and wonder why they do not get visits from their relatives.

The children mentioned what they would like their relatives to do for them. About 17.2 percent would like their relatives to continue helping them with food and schooling although they were under institutional care. Others (21 percent) suggested support in coping with the death of their parents. This could be in the form of visits, home stays and frequent contact. Others still (35 percent) would like their relatives to show them love and pray for them, give them hope and continue encouraging them in life as they would their own children.

Children and education

As observed, most of the children in this sub-sample are enrolled in school. Overall, all the children are happy to go to school. They pointed out that education will enable them to become somebody in life—they will shine in their careers, be independent, live a good life and help others. They also saw education as providing them with the knowledge and information that would be of benefit for the future. They indicated that education was essential—it will enable them to be productive in nation building. For many children (67 percent), school is like a second home. It is also a place where they met and interacted with friends. Negative feelings about school were also reported. Some children in the sub-sample children do not like school because they see it as stressful.

Children and goals for the future

Connected to education are the children's goals for the future. Indeed, the goals expressed were linked to careers and family life. Other related to national building. These are presented in Table 8.1.

Table 8.1 Children and goals

Goals for the future: Individual	Goals for the future: Communal
Have a family	Career in charitable/humanitarian organization
Be respected	Career in medicine/helping profession
Help the poor/sick	Career in legal field—child advocacy
Live a happy life	Career in education

Source: Created from our own data.

Children speak about human rights

Nearly all the children in the sub-sample from Nyumbani (95.7 percent) have heard of human rights. For them, human rights are privileges that everyone should have. All citizens of Kenya are entitled to these. To these children, these entitlements cannot be taken away by anyone, even one's own parents. To some, these rights guaranteed freedom and protection from mistreatment. Others still saw human rights as an opportunity—enabling the right holder to do what he/she wants to do. Children in the sub-sample looked at human rights as a demarcation of how a child should be treated—with respect and dignity.

Overall, the children felt that young people should have rights (93.6 percent). About half of these (48.9 percent) believe children should have the same rights as adults while another half (about 46.8 percent) feel children should not have the same rights as adults. Those who believe that children should have the same rights as adults, argued that adults and children are equal, hence should have the same rights. They pointed out that children are citizens of nations, they are not half-people; they are human beings and can make decisions on their own. To these children, everyone is "equal in God's eyes … whether male or female, young or old … everyone is equal." The group holding the opposite view indicated that adults and children are not the same—children are under age and cannot be treated like adults. If they were to be given same rights, some would abuse their freedoms and end up in trouble. Children are not well equipped to handle rights; they may be too explosive for them. This group felt that children should have their own set of rights that are appropriate for their age.

Children's view of the rights of the child

Although the children viewed all the rights as important, they highlighted some rights as instrumental to their welfare. These are presented in Figure 8.3.

The majority of the children (89.4 percent) reported that they enjoy most of the rights articulated in this chapter. Reactions varied regarding the children's views on who was responsible for enabling realizing their rights; 19.1 percent felt it was the duty of parents; 6.4 percent reported that the government was responsible for this; and 19.1 percent indicated that it was the community's responsibility. A considerable number (about 46.8 percent) were not sure who the primary duty bearer was.

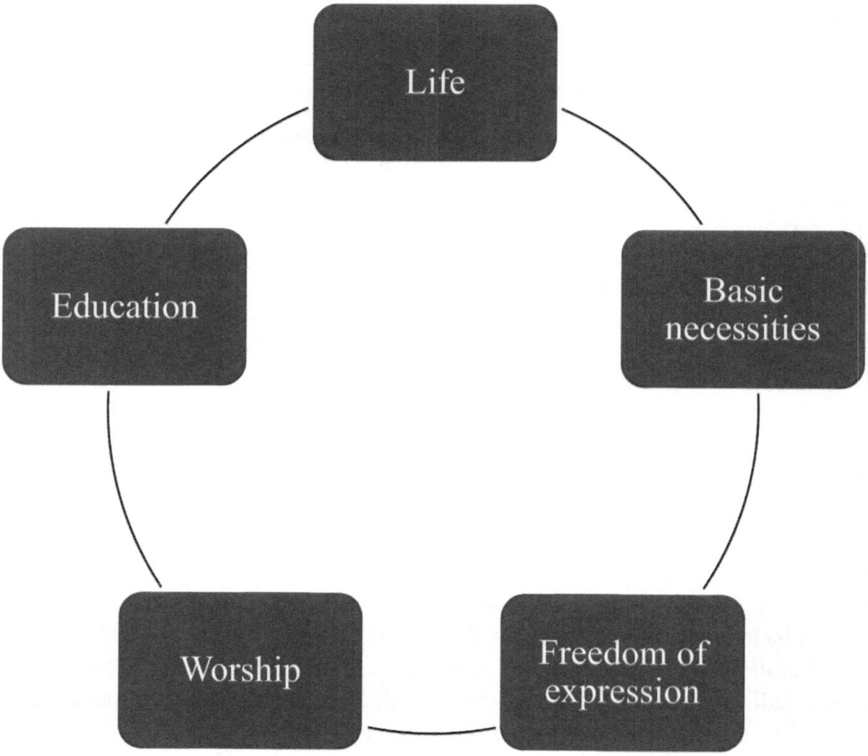

Figure 8.3 Rights considered important
Source: Authors' own data.

With respect to what should be done to promote awareness of children's rights, responses ranged from encouraging schools to play a key role in promoting these rights, making copies of the Children's Act available to all children in Kenya, and conducting public campaigns to ensure that adults including parents and other caregivers know the rights that are guaranteed to children.

With regard to ensuring that the rights of children are respected, the children suggested a number of actions. Primary among these was the need for advocacy mainly by children and allies like schools and caring adults, implementation of strict laws so that anyone in violation of children's rights is punished as well as creation of public space where children could talk about their rights.

Experiences of children in institutional care

Many of the children at Nyumbani Home (89.2 percent) reported being happy with their situation and living arrangements. Reasons given for their contentment focused on perception of love and acceptability. Other reasons given had to do with being taken care of and protected by parent figures. Still others dealt with the availability of basic necessities such as good food, a safe and clean environment, clothing, education and healthcare. The children also appreciate the fact that they have sponsors from other countries. The sense of togetherness they feel with other children in their situation was mentioned as important. In general, the children at the home are aware of children living on the street with little adult care, hence are grateful for what they have.

The children had many suggestions on what they would like to see happen in order to improve their living conditions at the home. These consisted of changing the menu (10 percent), giving children access to quality education by sending them to private schools (21 percent), and acknowledging the children's talents and abilities (18 percent). Other recommendations included encouraging interaction between older children and younger children so the children can have role models, encouraging visits from friends and relatives and introduction of time for leisure. There was also a sense, from some children, that nothing needed to change—life at the home was wonderful.

Children's voices on treatment of vulnerable children

In general, the children at the home reported being treated well by others—both adults and children. They also loved and respected each other. Some indicated that they were treated well at the home but not at school. Others pointed out that people's interactions with them changed when they learnt that they were HIV positive or that they lived at the home. Experiences of discrimination, especially at school, are not uncommon.

Generally, the perception is that people tend to show them love and kindness because they lived at the home. Alongside this, the children attributed the positive behavior towards them to individual traits like:

1. humility;
2. sincerity;
3. friendliness;
4. kindness;
5. trustworthiness.

With respect to how the children would like others to relate to them, the general feeling was that they would like to be treated like any other person—they would like to be loved, respected and treated with dignity. The majority of them (80 percent) would like others to relate to them with fairness, compassion and understanding. This, they believe, is how their own parents would behave towards them. They also argued that they are human and deserve to be treated with respect. The respondents also felt that they are children and did not choose to be HIV positive, hence should not be blamed for it.

What the children in the study sample would do to help other orphans and vulnerable children

With regards to what the respondents would do if they were in a position to help children classified as vulnerable, responses ranged from spiritual to material support. More specifically, the spiritual supported indicated include prayer and provision of hope for a better tomorrow. Material support indicated consisted of housing, clothing and food. Healthcare was also mentioned as one of the supports that the children would provide. Alongside this was effort to find a cure for HIV/AIDS. Strangely, some of the children reported that they will not be involved in supporting people infected with and/or affected by HIV/AIDS.

Nyumbani Village, Kutui, Kenya

Background

The Village was founded in 2006 and is part of the Children of God Relief Institute (COGRI). It seeks to be a self-sustaining, community-based residential village serving children orphaned as a result of HIV/AIDS. The model utilized involves placing children classified as OVC under the stewardship of an elderly grandparent figure. The concept of Nyumbani Village originated from the need to provide a family atmosphere for OVC under the care of an older relative, mostly a poor grandmother. In the village, children live together with their guardian as a family unit. This unit forms the basis for this discussion.

Demographic characteristics of the sub-sample

Many of the respondents at Nyumbani Village have been in either foster or institutional care most of their lives. The age was between 12 and 20, with the majority of the respondents falling within the 13–16 age range (80.4 percent). A significant component of the respondents were female (61.1 percent). Nearly all the respondents are currently attending school (95 percent). In fact, most of them are in primary school (83 percent). A significant proportion of the children in this sample (78 percent) reported being between the ages of 2 and 10 at the time of the death of their parent/s. All the respondents are orphans and reside at Nyumbani Village in Kitui, Kenya and have lived there for a considerable period of time (about four years).

Children and HIV/AIDS

All the children in this sub-sample have heard of AIDS. They perceive it to be a virus which has killed many people in Kenya. They point out that HIV/AIDS is a dangerous-killer disease without a cure, which can attack anybody. Although all the children at the Village have been somewhat affected by AIDS, a considerable number (70.7 percent) of the children did not know anyone who has AIDS. The children's relationship with AIDS-infected associates included family members such as fathers or brothers, cousins, friends and neighbors.

Children and the family (relationship with family members)

Most of the children at Nyumbani Village do not know the cause/s of their parents' death because they were relatively young at the time of the death of their parents. Factors associated with the death of their parents included TB, diabetes, typhoid, cancer, malaria, HIV/AIDS and meningitis. It is important to note that this information is based on recollection of what the children were told by members of the extended family.

When asked about their feelings with respect to the death of their parents, the children's reactions varied. Some (63.1 percent) reported feelings of sadness, sorrow and loneliness. Others (4.9 percent) reported feelings of resignation and prayed that God takes care of them. Few (about 7 percent) respondents expressed anger when they think of their parents. Others (24 percent) stated that although they felt aggrieved, they were grateful that they had found solace at Nyumbai Village. The reactions reported by the children concerning the death of their parent/s are presented in Figure 8.4.

Generally, the extended family is involved in the lives of children at Nyumbani Village. In fact, nearly all of them (97.6 percent) report being visited by a member of the extended family. During such visits, the children stated that they felt pleased, cared for, loved and comforted. To many of them, relatives represented their parents. The few who did not get any visits indicated feeling neglected; it was as though the extended family did not care whether or not they were dead or alive.

When asked how extended family relates to them, most of the children did not understand the question. Instead, they addressed the issue of what they would like the extended family to do for them. Suggestions included material assistance,

- Remember how happy they used to be when their parents were alive
- See other children with parents
- Feels that parents left them alone – uncared for
- Face problems like lack of food, shelter and other basic needs
- Cannot see their parents – miss them
- Loved their parents very much
- Cannot change the situation

Figure 8.4 Children's reaction to loss of parent/s

Source: Authors' own data.

guidance and advice. Other suggestion focused on love, acceptance and assistance with inheritance of property left by deceased parent/s.

Children and education

As observed earlier, all the respondents are currently in school. They all, without exception, indicated that school is important to them. They pointed out that education is the key to a better life. They felt school enabled them to gain knowledge and will open doors to prosperity. Besides this, they felt school was a place where they met new people and interacted with friends in a safe environment. Some see school as a place where they can read freely, something they enjoyed doing.

Children and goals for the future

Goals, for the majority of the children, are tied to education which they see as a means for the realization of their life plans. Aspirations of the children in the sub-sample were expressed mainly in career goals in the fields of education, medicine, nursing, commerce, military and health. Areas of interested also included engineering, driving and legal fields. The children feel, in the absence of parents, it was the duty of the Village and its administration to help the children attain their goals.

Children speak about human rights

Nearly all the children at Nyumbani Village (92.7 percent) have heard of human rights. To them, human rights mean a number of things. The main themes are listed in Table 8.2.

Table 8.2 Children's perceptions of human rights

Perceptions of human rights
Something a person is entitled to
Something a person has freedom to achieve
An entitlement recognized by everyone
Rights which person has to do something
Things that a person expects to be done for her/him
Things one should be given in life
They are things that one does freely

Source: Authors' own data.

All the children in the survey believe that children should have rights. In fact only a few of them (7.3 percent) indicated that children should not have the same rights as adults. These argued that adult have more life experience and can do much more than children can, hence deserve more rights. They also pointed out that adults are in a position to provide children with their rights and guide them.

Another argument advanced is that adults have more expectations placed on them, and as a result should have more rights than children. They children in this group felt this was not unjust because one day they will be adults and will enjoy adult rights then.

In terms of rights that they viewed as primary, about 97.6 percent of the children identified the following:

1. education;
2. basic needs and rights;
3. life;
4. worship;
5. leisure;
6. healthcare.

Many of the children in this sub-sample pointed out that they enjoy these rights.

The children indicated that it was the duty of society, including their community (39 percent), Nyumbani Village (26.8 percent) and adults (34.2 percent), to help them realize their rights. They also expressed the view that children could take action to ensure that their rights are realized. They saw being aware of their rights and advocacy as the starting point. They pointed out that Nyumbani Village, teachers and people in authority could play a major role in advocating for the rights of children and educating communities about these rights.

Ensuring that the rights of children were respected, protected and fulfilled, according to respondents, would require educating the children about their rights, ensuring that society respects guaranteed rights, and the empowerment of children as claim holders. We capture these perceptions in Figure 8.5.

Experiences of children in institutional care

All the children said that they are happy at the village. They stated that life was enjoyable, for the most part. Despite this observation, they made suggestions on what they would like to see improve in terms of their living situation.

The majority of the children in this sub-sample felt more attention should be devoted to encouraging the children to do well at school, have a positive attitude towards the institution, and themselves. They also expressed the need to engage more counselors and advisers. Other suggestions made related to the need to respect and obey the grandparents, creation of a more safe and clean environment as well as giving them opportunities for volunteering, especially in caring for the sick.

Children's voices on treatment of vulnerable children

Nearly all the respondents at Nyumbani Village reported being treated well (98.4 percent). They indicated that everyone, adults and children, were friendly and respectful. This could be because the village brought together children of similar characteristics under the care of nurturing adults. This assertion was

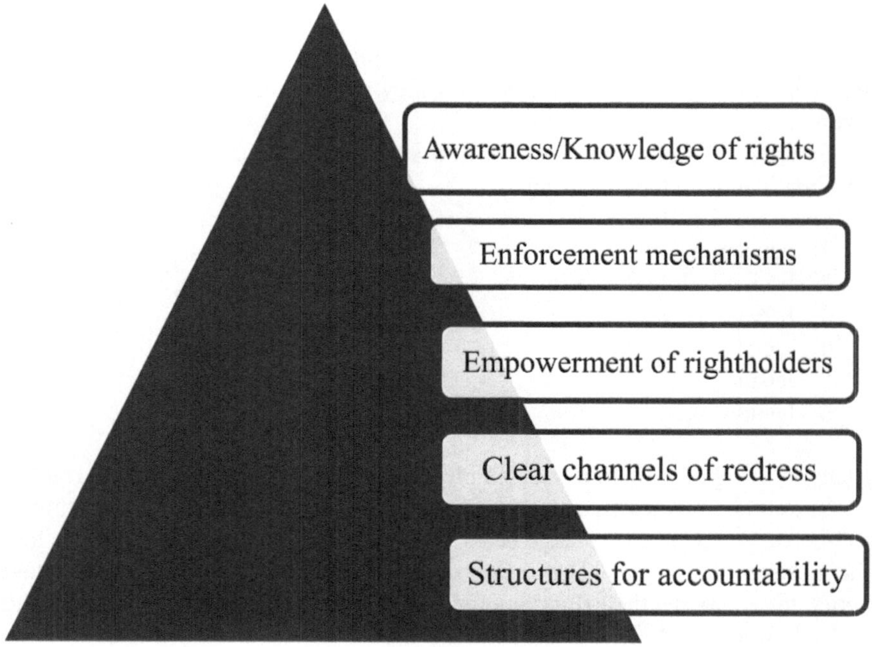

Figure 8.5 Process of rights attainment
Source: Authors' own data.

partially captured in the responses given by the children themselves. Indeed, the respondents felt that they shared a common bond (a common theme emerging was that they were all orphans and looked at each other as brothers and sisters)—they loved each other, played together, and did their chores together. They also reported that they were of good character, obedient and peaceful.

What the children in the study sample would do to help other orphans and vulnerable children

The children at Nyumbani Village expressed interest in supporting other children classified as vulnerable. Most of them would devote resources on educating vulnerable children, provision of quality healthcare along with basic necessities such as shelter, food and clothing. Others reported that they would volunteer to work with vulnerable children and show them love as well as support.

Conclusion

It is important to acknowledge the modest nature of the study conducted. Indeed, the study was exploratory and aimed at giving voice to the experiences of children classified as vulnerable. Due to data limitations, stringent statistical procedures could not be conducted. Another point of note is the small sample size, which limits ability to generalize lessons learned from the children in the study. Despite the observed limitations, the study was able to give the children an outlet to express their views about their experiences. One of the elements emphasized is the importance of education. The children see this as an avenue to a better future not only for themselves but also for their community. The children demonstrated sound understanding of human rights as these relate to the child. They, in addition, were able to identify parties responsible for ensuring that these rights are realized. These include governments, communities and schools. The children generally view adults as custodians of children's rights. In the context of sub-Saharan Africa, where children lack voice, realization of their rights might require authentic partnership with caring adults. This may be an important point in the journey of making children matter.

Globally, considerable effort has been devoted to the care of children classified as vulnerable. Despite this, examples abound to show that children considered vulnerable are not adequately provided for, even by governments that have ratified national and global instruments pertaining to the protection of children (UNAIDS et al., 2002; UNDP, 2012). In many instances, evidence suggests that budgetary commitments with regards to the welfare of children tend to be minimal or non-existent. Families and communities have been left to respond to the challenge with little assistance from governments. The heroism and generosity demonstrated, especially by women and communities of limited means, is commendable.

Civic organizations and anyone concerned about the welfare of children should stand together in holding governments accountable for the commitment they made to children through UNGASS and various agreements. Kenya and Zambia are among the countries that have developed and implemented national policies and strategies to strengthen capacities to manage the OVC crisis. There is hope that children classified as OVC will continue to have access to education, shelter, good nutrition, healthcare and other social services on an equal footing with other children. There is also hope that efforts to protect such children from abuse, violence, exploitation, discrimination, trafficking and loss of inheritance will continue, leading to attainment of their rights and realization of their full potential. After all, the future of these countries, and that of sub-Saharan Africa in general, rests on the shoulders of these children.

Bibliography

Care Kenya (2004). A Baseline Study on the Situation of Orphans and Vulnerable Children (OVC) in Kibera.

Foster, G. and Williamson, J. (2000). A review of current literature of the impact of HIV/AIDS on children in sub-Saharan Africa. *AIDS*, 14(suppl. 3), S275–S284.

UNAIDS, UNICEF and USAID (2002). Children on the Brink 2002: A Joint Report on Orphan Estimates and Program Strategies. Washington, DC: TvT Associates. http://www.unicef.org/media/publications/children_on_brink.pdf.
UNDP (2012). Global Commission on HIV and the Law (2012). HIV and the Law: Risks, Rights and Health. http://www.hivlawcommission.org/.

PART V
Making Children Matter

This section situates the discussion within the context of human rights. Specifically, it presents an overview of the situation of children in sub-Saharan Africa in relation to the Convention on the Rights of the Child (CRC). It also consolidates the key ideas articulated in the book. Key areas covered include: (1) the framework of the CRC and its historic evolution, its objectives and structure; (2) the meaning of the CRC to a vulnerable child in Africa; (3) the concept of OVC in Africa within the framework of the CRC; (4) challenges faced by OVC and how rights guaranteed under the convention may be realized by OVC; (5) a synthesis of the book's central ideas.

The section is organized under two distinct chapters. Chapter 9 locates OVC within the framework of the CRC. The book's concluding chapter, Chapter 10, deals with the key ideas examined in the book. A detailed overview of, and lessons learned from, each chapter is provided. The chapter closes with policy and program recommendations.

Chapter 9

Vulnerability among Children and the Convention on the Rights of the Child

Margaret Lombe and Harriet Mabikke

This chapter addresses the issue of vulnerability among children as this relates to the rights that are guaranteed under Convention on the Rights of the Child (CRC) and the extent to which these rights have been realized by children in sub-Saharan Africa. Specifically, the chapter presents a synopsis of the situation of vulnerable children and their experiences within the context of CRC. Key areas covered include:

1. the situation of vulnerable children in the region;
2. the framework of the Convention on the Rights of the Child and its historic evolution;
3. the meaning of the Convention on the Right of the Child to a vulnerable child in sub-Saharan Africa;
4. a review of mechanisms that may enhance attainment of rights guaranteed under CRC by OVC; and
5. an overview of why this discussion matters.

The chapter attempts to articulate the vulnerability experienced by OVC and its correlates including children's street living, child labor, trafficking in children, child soldiering and poverty. The authors review challenges children face in attaining their provision, protection and participation rights. Attention is given to show that while considerable progress has been made toward attainment of the rights guaranteed under the CRC, a lot still needs to be done to make these rights a reality for the African child.

The chapter touches on the concepts of convivencia and Ubuntu. The authors argue that OVC is a problematic terminology borne out of defective social institutions. The authors posit that the terminology, OVC, reflects the failure of social institutions to guarantee children rights that are primary to their wellbeing and healthy development. The term also stands in contradiction to familial and extra-familial systems of care that embody the African adage "it takes a village to raise a child." Indeed, the idea of community in which children matter—where every child belongs, is valued, loved and cared for—is refuted. The chapter closes with a reflection on why the CRC matters to children in sub-Saharan Africa, especially OVC.

Vulnerability among Children in Sub-Saharan Africa: An Overview

The high prevalence of HIV/AIDS in sub-Saharan Africa has resulted in a dramatic increase in orphans and vulnerable children (OVC) over the past decade (Lombe and Ochumbo, 2008). Vulnerability among children now appears to be a permanent feature of the region. Most recent data show that, at the end of 2010, an estimated 16.6 million children had lost one or both parents to HIV/AIDS worldwide; 14.9 million of these (89.8 percent) reside in sub-Saharan Africa. This number represents more than a two-fold increase in the number of orphans since 2000 (UNICEF, 2011b). Evidence exists to suggest that orphaned children typically rely on extended familial networks for support. However, the magnitude of the crisis has overwhelmed traditional familial networks of care, diminishing the capacity to care for economically and socially vulnerable children (Lombe and Ochumbo, 2008; Ssewamala et al., 2010). The HIV/AIDS pandemic has also diminished the human capital of families through adult mortality as well as the ability of households to generate resources diverted toward caregiving (McPherson, 2005). This phenomenon has placed orphaned and other vulnerable children at increased danger of risk factors including sexual risk-taking, reduced access to healthcare, increased psychosocial adversity and dropping out of school. Children in this group also suffer from discrimination and stigma. As observed, a growing number of children in this group are to be found in child-headed households, further heightening their vulnerability.

Despite the noted vulnerability, only about 10–25 percent of affected children receive any type of external assistance (Horton and Das, 2008; UNICEF, 2011b). Further, much of the assistance given has focused primarily on provision of basic necessities to vulnerable children and their households. Limited attention has been devoted to interventions with long-lasting effects. Moreover, effort currently in place put little emphasis on attainment of the rights guaranteed under the CRC, despite the fact that realization of the rights allowed under CRC may be important for children to realize their full potential free from hunger, want, neglect and abuse. We acknowledge the fact that issues facing vulnerable children in sub-Saharan Africa are numerous and complex. Indeed, multifaceted approaches may be needed to respond to this intricate phenomenon. In this chapter, we focus only on vulnerability as this relates to human rights as guaranteed under the CRC and the extent to which these rights have been realized by children in sub-Saharan Africa.

Convention on the Rights of the Child: Historical Evolution, Structure and Objectives

The Convention on the Right of the Child was adopted and opened for signature, ratification and accession by General Assembly resolution 44/25 in November 1989 and entered into force in 1990. It is important to note that UN member states, in principle, UN member countries, collectively recognized the rights of children in the Universal Declaration of Human Rights, through a non-binding resolution adopted by the UN General Assembly in 1948 (UN, n.d.). The Declaration states, "Motherhood and childhood are entitled to special care and assistance. All children, whether born in or out of wedlock, shall enjoy the same social protection." UN member states further enunciated children's rights by unanimously adopting the Declaration on the Rights of the Child in 1959 (Walther, 2003). This Declaration, which incorporated language from the Universal Declaration of Human Rights, called on governments, families and individuals to ensure that all children everywhere enjoyed certain rights, including the right to appropriate legal protections, a name and nationality, access to healthcare, and protection from abuse and exploitation. The international community also acknowledged the special rights of children in the International Covenant on Economic, Social, and Cultural Rights (CESCR) and the International Covenant on Civil and Political Rights (CCPR), which entered into force in 1976 (WHO, n.d.; UNHCR, 2011).

Although the principles outlined in the International Bill of Rights apply to all humans including children, the Convention on the Rights of the Child articulates the rights that children are entitled to more completely and provides a set of guiding principles that fundamentally shapes the way in which society views and responds to children. The possibility of a Convention on the Rights of the Child was first raised by the government of Poland in 1978 as UN member states planned activities and programs that would be executed during the calendar year 1979; a year designated by UN member states as the International Year of the Child (Jupp, 1990; UNICEF, 1990). For a decade following this, UN member states participated in a UN Commission on Human Rights (now the Human Rights Council), a working group charged with the task of drafting the text of the CRC. The Convention was adopted by the UN General Assembly in 1989 after a decade of deliberations.

The Convention sets out the necessary environment and means to enable every child to develop and realize their full potential. In addition to laying the foundational principles from which all rights—in relation to the child—must be achieved, the Convention calls for the provision of specific resources, skills and contributions necessary to ensure the survival and development of children to their maximum capability. The rights guaranteed under the CRC are contained in 54 articles and establish steps to protect children from hunger, want, neglect, exploitation and abuse (see Table 7.3 for a summary of the CRC). The articles on the Convention on the Rights of the Child are organized around four categories as follows:

1. Guiding principle—based on non-discrimination and adherence to the best interest of the child.
2. Survival and development rights—focusing on rights to resources, skills and other factors necessary for the survival and full development of the child.

3. Protection rights—recognition that society has a responsibility to protect children from all forms of abuse, neglect, exploitation and cruelty.
4. Participation rights—focusing on the freedom of the child to have a say in decisions that affect their socio-economic, religious, political life, right to information and to participate in decision-making.

In a sense the Convention puts the limelight on the child and helps define a child. It also stresses the fact that the rights of the child are not special rights but human rights which every child is entitled to. The CRC acknowledges that children start life dependent, hence are uniquely positioned and entitled to special protection. It also recognizes the child as an individual despite the fact that he or she is a member of a family and community. The CRC also acknowledges the child's responsibilities to her family, community and society, but these are to be appropriate for her own age. This is also recognition of the fact that children lack voice, and the capacity to advocate on their own behalf. Indeed, action or inaction of government often has a disproportional and at times negative impact on children more than any other group/s. In this way the child is acknowledged as a right holder, a subject of its own rights—and not an object of charity. The duty-bearer is set aside as the parents and state, at the legal level, and society, at the moral level.

As of December 2010, the Convention had been ratified by all but two countries—the United States and Somalia. The near-universal ratification of the Convention reflects a global commitment to the principles of children's rights. By ratifying the Convention, governments express their commitment to avail, protect and guarantee the rights assured under the CRC. State parties are obligated to amend and create laws and policies to fully implement the Convention; they are required to consider all actions taken in light of the best interests of the child. The task, however, may require allegiance from all; society is a duty-bearer to the world's children. Indeed, the standards and principles articulated in the Convention can only become a reality when they are respected by everyone—the family, school system and other social institutions. Society has a stake in ensuring the healthy development of children—as the adage goes, "children are our future."

The CRC and Concept of OVC in Sub-Saharan Africa: A Problematic Discourse

The term Orphans and Vulnerable Children (OVC) generally refers to orphans and other groups of children who are at high risk of exposure to social and environmental threats. Operationally, OVC defines a group of children who experience negative outcomes, such as loss of education, morbidity and malnutrition, at higher rates compared to their peers (ACPF, 2008, 2011). The children in this group need special attention to facilitate their participation in society at levels that are appropriate for their age. It's important to underscore the fact that children, by default, are inherently vulnerable. They depend on adults for their physical, emotional and developmental needs. However, children characterized as OVC are more vulnerable due to "additional circumstances which aggravate their exposure to risk" (Liebenberg, 2010: 230). According to the UNAIDS report 2010, OVC are more likely to suffer from malnutrition, to become street children and engage in sexual activity before the age of 15. They are also less likely to attend school compared to children who live with at least one parent. Going by this definition, the concept of OVC by and in itself reflects a problematic discourse. Indeed, defining children as vulnerable stands in stark contradiction with the CRC in that it's an acknowledgment of a societal failure to fulfill its obligation to the right holder—the children. Undeniably, that some children can still be categorized as vulnerable more than 20 years after the CRC came into force with near-universal ratification from all UN member states highlights this contradiction. As observed in the foregoing discussion, by ratifying the CRC, states, including governments of African countries, committed themselves to abide by the four core principles of the Covenant: non-discrimination; devotion to the best interests of the child; the right to life, survival and development; and respect for the views of the child. Further, in addition to the CRC, the African Union, in an effort to augment the CRC and embrace social-cultural and economic realities that are inherently African with respect to children's rights, adopted the African Charter on the Rights and Welfare of the Child (ACRWC or the Children's Charter), which has been ratified by 45 of the 53 African countries (UNHCR, 2011). As has been observed by others (see, e.g., UNHCR, 2011), the Children's Charter emerged out of the sentiment that the CRC ignored some vital socio-cultural and economic realities of the African child. Such realities included, among others, the different definitions of a child, a child's role in the family and community as well as the question of addressing harmful practices such as female genital mutilation.

Despite the existence of the two instruments that clearly spell out the rights of children, and the significant proportion of children globally (children make up about 40 percent of the population of sub-Saharan Africa), considerable numbers of children in sub-Saharan Africa continue to be denied their human rights, compromising their life chances. Indeed, children continue to experience unimaginable hardships; they are denied the right to a safe childhood, education and leisure. In certain cases they are forced into marriages, engaged as child soldiers, forced to live on streets, and experience hunger and other abuses.

Vulnerabilities among children have become a permanent feature of the landscape of sub-Saharan Africa. The region has the highest number of OVC worldwide, about 9 in 10 OVC live in this region (UNAIDS, 2008). In addition, countries characterized as hyper-endemic HIV epidemics, where prevalence rates surpass 15 percent of the general population aged 15–49, are to be found in sub-Saharan Africa (UNAIDS, 2009). As is the case with many concepts, definitions of vulnerability vary considerably in sub-Saharan African. In most of these countries, however, vulnerable children encompass children affected/infected by HIV/AIDS, orphaned children, street children, children living in households headed by a child, child laborers, children with disabilities, and sexually exploited children. Vulnerable children also include those affected by armed conflict, children in impoverished households, refugees and displaced children, those that are neglected, destitute or abandoned, and those who have a terminally ill parent or guardian along with children at risk of other abuses. It should be acknowledged that differences in definition may exist across countries. However, despite these differences, the underlying theme is the idea that children in this group are defenseless, unprotected, exposed to physical and emotional harm. They are vulnerable to poor health and malnutrition, to lack of schooling, to lack of rest and leisure, to being forced into armed forces, to injury both physical and mental, among others; all in violation of their rights as set forth in the different articles of the CRC. A brief overview of key articles follows.

Article 6 of the CRC guarantees every child an inherent right to life. It is the responsibility of governments and other duty-bearers including parents and society to ensure that children thrive and live healthy lives. Article 24 further guarantees children the right to good healthcare both in terms of access and quality. According to this Article, children have a right to the enjoyment of the highest attainable standard of health. Toward this, the CRC urges governments to diminish child and infant mortality, to ensure pre- and post-natal care, combat disease and malnutrition and abolish traditional practices that are detrimental to children's health.

In spite of these and related articles, health is one of the areas in which children in sub-Saharan Africa continue to be especially vulnerable. Sub-Saharan Africa has the highest rates of infant mortality in the world. In 2008, one in seven children in this region died before the age of five; representing half of all child deaths worldwide (HIV Global Report, 2010). Despite advances made in the medical field, death from preventable diseases, such as malaria and AIDS-related complications, persist among children. In general, although many of the children in sub-Saharan African are at risk of being denied the right to life and good health, children classified as OVC, are perhaps the group that faces the greatest risk. Indeed, for the most part, children affected by HIV and AIDS are at a higher risk of being affected by HIV themselves. Existing data suggests that children in this group are more at risk of HIV infection compared to other children. Due to lack of parental care and supervision as well as socio-economic pressure, they are more likely to become sexually active at a younger age; making them more susceptible to infection. Moreover, some children in this group may have been born with HIV through mother-to-child transmission (UNAIDS, 2009).

It has to be acknowledged that current trends suggest that HIV infections and AIDS-related deaths among children are declining. This is welcome news. Moreover, according to the HIV Global Report (2010), provision of antiretroviral (ARV) drugs to prevent mother-to-child HIV transmission has risen by 15 percent between 2005 and 2009. Although children's access to antiretroviral therapy has gone up substantially in recent years, data from UNICEF (2009) indicates that only 28 percent of the estimated 1.27 million children needing antiretroviral therapy worldwide were able to receive it during the year 2009. Further, in Eastern and Southern Africa, the locality most severely affected by the epidemic, only 32 percent of these children received ARVs. This figure is unacceptably low.

Children's rights to a healthy life are further compromised by governments' failure to eradicate harmful traditional practices such as Female Genital Mutilation/ Cutting (FGM/C). FGM/C may be seen as a fundamental violation of Article 24 of the CRC that specifically compels governments to abolish traditional practices that are detrimental to children's health. According to this Article, children should be protected from all forms of violence, injury or abuse. Mali, Ivory Coast, Benin, Niger, Sudan, Eritrea, Ethiopia, Kenya and Tanzania are among the countries in sub-Saharan Africa that have a high prevalence of FGM/C (UNICEF, 2013).

Children's lives are further put at risk by their recruitment into armed forces. Worldwide, an estimated 300,000 children are engaged in armed conflicts in violation of Article 38 of the CRC. Moreover, a considerable number of governments in sub-Saharan Africa are known to have recruited children into armed forces (ILO, 2003). Such countries include: Angola, Burundi, Central African Republic, Cote d'Ivoire, Chad, Democratic Republic of Congo, Guinea, Liberia, Rwanda, Sierra Leone, Somalia and Uganda. Article 38 of the CRC urges governments to take all feasible measures to ensure that children under the age of 15 are not directly engaged in hostilities and are not recruited into armed forces. In addition, although the Optional Protocol on the involvement of children in armed forces sets the age of 15 as the age at which children can enlist in armed forces, it requires governments to "take all feasible measures" to ensure that members of the armed forces under the age of 18 do not take a direct part in hostilities. The very idea of child soldiers is contrary to the principle of CRC. Involvement of children in hostilities does not only expose them to harm, it also has the potential to compromise their life chances. Children characterized as OVC may be especially at risk because of their already vulnerable situation. Another group at risk is girls. Indeed, many of the child soldiers are girls who are vulnerable to sexual victimization, to being raped and to being given to military commanders as "wives." This is evident in the case of the Lord's Resistance Army in northern Uganda, where girls have been known to be exploited for sex, making them vulnerable to HIV infection. The fact that children continue to be seized and used as "soldier wives" for rebels may be interpreted as a clear failure on the part of states and the international community as duty-bearers to safeguard the rights of the child. Specifically, the child's right not be recruited into armed forces, protection of its best interests, its right to life, to health, to an education, its right to rest and leisure and above all the child's right to protection against all forms of violence as set forth in Article 19 of the CRC.

Article 28 of the CRC guarantees children the right to an education. Among others, this Article requires governments to make primary education free and available to all children, regardless of socio-economic status. The Article compels governments to encourage young people to attain the highest level of education dictated by their capabilities. The Article also obliges governments to encourage attendance and reduce school dropouts as well as to regulate disciplinary procedures so that these are conducted in a way that respects the dignity of the child.

The AIDS pandemic has greatly affected the rights of children in sub-Saharan Africa, including their right to an education. Undeniably, the impact of the AIDS pandemic on children's rights to an education—especially OVC—cannot be overstated. In fact, research evidence exists to suggest that OVC are less likely to be enrolled in school and are more likely to drop out of school compared to children living with both parents and/or those with at least one parent (UNICEF, 2009). In Uganda, for instance, amongst children aged 15–19 years whose parents had died, only 29 percent continued their schooling undisrupted; 25 percent lost school time and 45 percent dropped out of school completely (Sengendo and Nambi, 1997; UNICEF, 2009). Even when in school, orphaned children are less likely to concentrate on studies than non-orphaned children and are therefore more likely to have a poor performance due to their situations. Furthermore, orphans and other vulnerable children are at higher risk of missing out on schooling and the protective cushion that schooling provides; they are therefore more likely to be exposed to HIV, sustaining the cycle of infection. This is especially true in the case of girls. Although similar numbers of girls and boys start schooling, boys from vulnerable backgrounds are more likely to complete primary education compared to their female counterparts. Of the estimated 30 million children out of school, 53 percent are girls (UNICEF, 2010). As indicated by research evidence, keeping girls in school may have positive externalities such as optimistic orientation toward the future, reduced vulnerability and increased employability. It may also provide a buffer to HIV/AIDS risk.

Moreover, the rights of OVC to education have been further confounded by the fact that females are disproportionately impacted by HIV in sub-Saharan Africa. According to UNAIDS (2010), 76 percent of all HIV-positive women in the world live in this region. This has had a significant impact on children's abilities to claim their right to an education. Anecdotal evidence suggests that compared to men, women tend to make better choices with respect to their children's education and health. The absence of women in the lives of children may exacerbate their chances of getting an education. In addition, AIDS has challenged the capacity and quality of educational systems across sub-Saharan Africa. Evidence indicates that AIDS continues to kill working-age adults faster than they can be replaced. This also holds true for persons in the profession of teaching. In the case of Zambia, for instance, an estimated 815 primary school teachers died from AIDS in 2000, representing 45 percent of all teachers trained that year (Germann et al., 2009).

Children have a right to rest and enjoy leisure according to Articles 31 and 32 of the CRC. Article 31 compels governments to recognize the right of the child to rest and leisure and to engage in play and recreational activities. Article 32 among others guarantees children a right to protection from economic exploitation and from performing any work that interferes with the child's education and is harmful to the child's health. In many parts of sub-Saharan Africa, children are generally expected to engage in productive activities such as performing household chores and taking care of younger siblings. Moreover, mainly due to raising levels of poverty and food insecurity, children are increasingly being driven into the labor market. The majority of these are to be found in the secondary labor market, characterized by low wages and poor working conditions. According to UNICEF (2009), a third of the children between the ages of 5 and 14 in sub-Saharan Africa were workers in 2008. OVC are especially at higher risk of being drawn into the labor market at younger ages. They work mostly as domestic help; making them susceptible to abuse and sexual exploitation. In Tanzania, mainly because of their smaller bodies and dexterity, children are forced to work in mines harvesting the valuable mineral tanzanite, facing possibilities of injuries, disease and even death. Countries with high numbers of child laborers include: Chad (53 percent of all children), Ethiopia (53 percent), Somalia (49 percent), Sierra Leone (48 percent) and Burkina Faso (47 percent) (ILO, 2013).

Articles 11 and 35 speak against kidnapping, abduction, sale and trafficking of children. The provisions in the Convention are further augmented by the Optional Protocol on the sale of children, child prostitution and child pornography. These treaties urge governments to take measures to ensure that children are protected from such atrocities. Despite the stipulations alluded to in the foregoing discussion, children in sub-Saharan Africa remain at risk of falling prey to human traffickers and are at risk of being traded for sexual exploitation, organ harvesting, labor and other forms of exploitation (Toepfer and Wells, cited in Roby, 2005). Current estimates are that about 1.2 million women and children enter the global commercial sex market every year (UNDP, 2003).

OVC, in particular, are at higher risk of falling victim to human trafficking because of their vulnerable situation and the high rates of poverty that characterize such households. Further, due to ineffective civil society and civil institutions, in many countries of sub-Saharan Africa, proper accountability for and protection of children is rarely undertaken, making it easier for traffickers to navigate the system. Furthermore, increased interaction among countries triggered by globalization has introduced new levels of consumerism and classification of indigenous people as a commodity. In many African countries, females and children are treated as property and virtually exploited not just by society but by their immediate families, hence, it comes as no surprise that while families may lose children to abduction, others make the decision to sell their offspring for economic gains. Coupled with this is the belief, which is prominent in many parts of sub-Saharan Africa, that having sexual intercourse with a virgin "has restorative or healing powers" (Roby, 2005). This, in fact, has fueled the demand for young girls exponentially. Addressing the issue of human trafficking, especially as it affects children, is especially arduous not only because of the difficulty of redressing the micro and macro factors that lead to its potency but also because the implementation of policies that curb and eventually eliminate the problem is thwarted by widespread corruption. Further, OVC often lack supervision and therefore easily fall into the cracks of social systems and treaties that protect other children.

Furthermore, children, OVC in particular, continue to bear the cost of poorly articulated policies and cultural practices. Indeed, in many parts of sub-Saharan Africa, some provisions of customary law negatively impact the child. In matters of inheritance, for example, there is a tendency by relatives of an intestate to rely on the customary practice of denying children their inheritance. Children are often left to suffer from the emotional trauma associated with property grabbing upon loss of a parent/s. Further, the marriage age, as defined by customary law, is not well defined in many parts of sub-Saharan Africa, leaving children, especially young girls, at the mercy of relatives. It should be noted that, for the most part, laws that are designed to safeguard the welfare of the child exist. However, these are often poorly articulated. Further, the process of litigation is slow and inefficient and, in many cases, redress may come too late. Moreover, children are not even aware of the laws and their own rights. Also, they may not even fully understand the process of redress. This, it should be noted, occurs despite provisions articulated under Articles 4 and 42 of CRC which mandates governments to make the Convention known to adults and children.

OVC as Challenge to the Concepts of Convivencia, and "Ubuntu" and the Familial Systems of Care

As noted, children in many parts of the world make up about half of the population yet they continue to be insecure worldwide. Children make up a significant proportion of people in poverty, groups at risk of dying from preventable diseases, and are subjected to justice systems that, for the most part, do not even recognize their special needs. This is despite the existence of rights that are guaranteed under the CRC. In this section we attempt to explore the concept of OVC and how this relates to convivencia and/or Ubuntu.

The idea of OVC stands in unadulterated contradiction to the notion of convivencia; the concept of "Ubuntu" and the familial systems of care. Convivencia is the idea of personhood that defines humans, regardless of social standing, as creative agents with capacity to influence their life circumstances (Lombe, 2008). "Ubuntu" emphasizes the interconnectedness of humans—the idea that "my humanity is connected to yours; as such neither of us can survive without the other." According to Archbishop Desmond Tutu, Ubuntu is at the center of human existence and it is reflected in the "I am what I am because of who we all are. I am because you are."

> 'Ubuntu' is the essence of being human. It speaks of the fact that my humanity is caught up and is inextricably bound up in yours. I am human because I belong. It speaks about humaneness, gentleness, hospitality, putting yourself out on behalf of others, being vulnerable. It embraces compassion and toughness. It recognizes that my humanity is bound up in yours, for we can only be human together. (Bhengu, 2006)

Reflecting on these two concepts, it becomes fundamentally wrong and unjust to classify children as vulnerable and leave them to lead susceptible lives, excluded from aspects of citizenship enjoyed by others. Indeed, our humanity, as conceived under the lenses of Ubuntu, demands that we care for each other; more so, for the weaker members of the human family, including children. The term OVC indicates a major breakdown in the communal/societal systems of care. AIDS has so strained the familial systems of care that the concept of "Ubuntu" with regards to children has been tested. Prior to the AIDS epidemic, in many parts of Africa, the concept of "orphan" or "vulnerable child" was non-existent; children belonged not only to the biological mother and father but to the whole community. It indeed took a village to raise a child! Every capable adult within a community, invested somewhat in the wellbeing of the child. Adults provided guidance, they nurtured and corrected. Since the rearing of the child was a communal affair, children did not have to fend for themselves; they were naturally absorbed by the communal systems of care. Largely due to the AIDS pandemic and the staggering numbers of AIDS related orphans, coupled with the loss of working-age adults, the familial and other social networks that absorbed orphans have been severely strained. The strain has also been exacerbated by relentless bouts of poverty that characterize the region. AIDS has shattered "Ubuntuism" in many African communities, making OVC even more vulnerable: as observed, they are in danger of sexual advances/ exploitation, even from family members, victims of land grabbing, and the "sugar daddy" phenomenon as well as many other social evils which society protected children from prior to the proliferation of the AIDS epidemic.

With the abdication of its responsibility to nurture and protect its children, society has lost the moral authority to guide. Indeed, the social fabric that holds peoples together has been compromised. In the long run, society bears the cost of failing children. Society pays in the cost of reduced capacity, the cost of failure of children to attain their full potential and contribute to society in a meaningful way, the cost of squandered potential to positively impact economic productivity and the price of loss of voice, politically. On the other hand, strengthening both familial and extra-familial systems of care may produce positive externalities. These may accrue to the individual child, community and society. Benefits to the child may include the sense of security that comes from being protected, cared for and valued. They may also consist of feeling part of the whole—sense of belonging, sense of obligation to the community, empowerment, positive orientation and enhanced dignity as well as self-worth. Benefits that may accrue to the community include building communal trust, validating or strengthening local systems of care, strengthening local networks, solidarity and interrelatedness. Societal benefits may include creation of communities of stakeholders, enhancing capacity to protect children and development of social cohesion.

Does the African Child Understand the CRC? Does the Child Understand its Role as a Right-Holder?

Extensive research has been conducted with respect to OVC. Most of this, however, has focused on addressing the immediate physical needs of OVC. This is commendable give the magnitude of vulnerability experienced by children in this category. What may be problematic, however, is the fact that little attention has been undertaken to look at the issue of OVC from a rights-based perspective, through the prism of the CRC. Little information exist with regards to whether or not children termed OVC, especially in sub-Saharan Africa, are even aware of the existence of the CRC. Given the lack of data on the subject, we draw mainly from the study conducted with children from Kenya and Zambia.

As rights-holders, children have a valid claim to rights such as education, health, protection and leisure, among others. They are subjects of their rights with potential to make a claim. Governments, as duty-bearers, have a direct responsibility to ensure that children are empowered with the knowledge and skills to enable them make a claim on rights guaranteed under the CRC. Oftentimes, however, children are portrayed as vulnerable beings in need of charity. Their views are rarely heard or considered in the political process or even on issues that directly affect them. In many parts of sub-Saharan Africa, cultural practices encourage submissive disposition from children, especially in relation to authority figures, stifling their voices and capacity to contribute to society. Moreover, the idea that "children should be seen and not heard from," which is common in many parts of Africa, further inhibits the capacity of children to act as agents with potential to influence outcomes in their favour.

The lack of meaningful participation that characterizes children stands as a major obstacle to their attainment of rights warranted under the CRC. Realization of these rights may require a meaningful cultural shift. A shift that allows for significant change of social norms to occur; creating space for children to have a voice and engage meaningfully in matters that affect them. This may require more than token participation, such as is displayed on the Day of the African Child (DAC), celebrated every year on June 16, when the African child is seen reciting poems, often written for her by adults. The voice of the African child may need to be strengthened so it can be heard on issues affecting children, including birth registrations, violence against children, education and child trafficking, to mention a few.

Enhancing the Child's Capacity to Attain Rights Guaranteed Under the CRC

For children to be able to claim their provision, protection and participation rights, they need to be aware the existence of these rights in the first place. In this regard, the primary responsibility of governments and other duty-bearers is to educate children on the rights warranted by the CRC. Moreover, this effort should include educating children on the role as right-holders endowed with the capacity to make a claim. Given that children are members of families and communities, in addition to educating children about their rights, emphasis should be put on instructing parents and other members of the community about their role as duty-bearers along with what this entails in regards to children.

Headway has been made with respect to safeguarding the rights of the child in sub-Saharan Africa. In the past decade many African governments have aligned their national legislations with international and/or regional treaties, e.g., the CRC and the African Charter on the Rights and Welfare of the Child, by incorporating children's rights into their constitution, laws and policies. Pertaining to education, considerable advances have been made. For example, Senegal, in 2000, implemented the Education for All Act, expanding the provision of basic. Gender parity in education has also been greatly enhanced through the introduction of the Universal Primary Education (UPE) initiative in many countries in Africa, including Lesotho, Kenya, Ethiopia, Mozambique and Uganda. Despite these gains, challenges still exist in addressing children's rights as they relate to education. As stipulated under the CRC, the right to education encompasses both quality and accessibility. In many parts of sub-Saharan Africa, both quality and access continue to be problematic. Indeed, the UPE initiative, good as it is, was implemented as a requirement to trigger realization of the second of the Millennium Development Goals—provision of universal primary education. In many countries the UPE initiative was implemented without investing in the infrastructure (e.g., schools and teachers) necessary to support the initiative. As a result, the initiative has challenged the capacity of the educational system to cope with the increasing demands; compromising the quality of the free primary education. Access to education has been further confounded by the demand for a user fee, required for enrollment in primary schools. Children in families that are unable to meet this requirement have no safety net, hence are denied the opportunity to enroll and complete basic primary.

Further, it is common knowledge that children, especially in rural areas, have to walk extensive distances to get to school. In fact, prohibitive distances are said to limit school attendance for younger children and girls. Furthermore, the quality of education provided, in some parts of the region, leaves a lot to be desired. Education, for the most part, is based on the pedagogy of memorization at the expense of critical thinking. Coupled with this is the shortage of teachers as well as teaching material. Further, where teachers are available, they are often underpaid. In addition, children in this region generally do not understand that quality and accessible education is their right, something that they are entitled to. Moreover, they lack the capacity to make a claim. Also, the mechanism of redress is not well articulated to allow for the right-holder to make a claim.

Conclusion: Why the CRC Matters to OVC and Other Children

The Convention on the Rights of the Child is one of the most ambitious policy undertakings at the global level. It places the child at the center and underscores the importance of the child in the discourse of human rights. It is also a representation of the promise the global community makes to the world's children and its commitment to enable children to realize the rights guaranteed under the CRC. It bids everyone to pay attention to specific aspects of the child's life and to treat the child with respect and dignity. It underscores the fact that all children deserve to be protected and to be given the best possible chance in life simply because they're children.

The Convention clearly outlines the right-holder and defines duty-bearers. By so doing, it creates a new vision of the child and brings together different provisions aimed at protecting the child through positive action by primary stakeholders, including the child's country, parents and relevant institutions. It also recognizes the child as a holder of participatory rights and freedoms, while stressing the country's duty to help families care for and protect the child.

The Convention is important to all children, especially OVC, in that it empowers the child to think and act proactively as an agent endowed with capacity to influence outcomes in its favor. Indeed, when the child appreciates its position as a right-holder, it learns to engage with the world differently and the world responds accordingly. Agency empowers the child to understand its potential to shape its destiny. An appreciation of the state of agency has the potential to enable the child to engage the world with boldness—the child has a stake in its future. Outward-looking children are excited about their future and prospects; they are hopeful children and have the ability to dream and attain their dreams, thus empowering the child to lose the servitude/submissive attitude. This all starts with knowledge and appreciation of the rights guaranteed to the child under the CRC, in a sense the CRC provides a framework for agency.

The Convention is an important tool in advocating for the needs of children around the world. Indeed, its principles are applied in regular programming of many NGOs and humanitarian agencies whose work focuses on addressing the needs of children. Armed with the CRC, these institutions are empowered to hold duty-bearers accountable.

The CRC can be seen as an assessment tool for governments and other duty-bearers in evaluating progress in meeting children's needs. The Convention may be applied as a shaming tool with respect to governments who have reneged on their promises to children. The CRC provides a moral compass for the world in its engagement with children. It is used as a yardstick to measure how the world has performed in protecting the dignity of the child.

In the hands of children, the CRC is a powerful advocacy tool enabling children demand and realize their rights. Indeed, as they engage with societal institutions such as parents, governments, and schools, they come from an informed perspective. For example, a child who understands its right to leisure would boldly demand this right when it's not readily availed. Because the CRC exists, the world is forced to look at children not as objects of charity and pity, but rather as subjects of their own rights.

Bibliography

African Child Policy Forum (ACPF) (2008). In the best interests of the child: Harmonising laws on children in Eastern and Southern Africa. http://www.africanchildinfo.net.

African Child Policy Forum (ACPF) (2011). In the best interests of the child: Harmonising laws on children in West and Central Africa. http://www.africanchildinfo.net.

Bhengu, M.J. (2006). *Ubuntu: The Global Philosophy for Humankind.* Cape Town: Lotsha Publications.

Germann, S., Ngoma, F., Wamimbi, R., et al. (2009). Mobilizing and strengthening community-led childcare through community care groups and coalitions: A study from Ethiopia, Mozambique, Uganda and Zambia. *International NGO Journal*, 4(1), 1–6.

HIV Global Report (2010). The global AIDS epidemic 2010. http://www.unaids.org/globalreport/Global_report.htm.

Horton, R. and Das, P. (2008). Putting prevention at the forefront of HIV/AIDS. *Lancet*, 372, 421–2.

International Labor Organization (ILO) (2003). http://www.ilo.org/wcmsp5/groups/public/@ed_emp/@emp_ent/@ifp_crisis/documents/publication/wcms_116566.pdf.

International Labor Organization (ILO) (2013). Global child labor trends 2008–2010. http://www.ilo.org/ipec/Informationresources/lang--en/index.htm.

Jupp, M. (1990). The UN Convention on the Rights of the Child: An Opportunity for Advocates. *Human Rights Quarterly*, 12(1), 130–36.

Liebenberg, S. (2010). *Socio-economic Right: Adjudication Under a Transformative Constitution.* Cape Town: Juta Law.

Lombe, M. and Ochumbo, A. (2008). Sub-Saharan Africa's orphan crisis: Challenges and opportunities. *International Social Work*, 51, 682–98.

Lombe, M. and Sherraden, M. (2008). Effects of participating in an asset-building intervention on social inclusion. *Journal of Poverty*, 12(3), 284–305.

MCDSS and GTZ (Ministry of Community Development and Social Services, Government of Zambia and German Technical Cooperation) (2006). *Monitoring Report 2nd Edition: Pilot Social Cash Transfer Scheme, Kalomo District, Zambia*. Lusaka: Author.

McPherson, M.F. (2005). Asset preservation in African agriculture in the face of HIV/AIDS: The role of education. *American Journal of Agricultural Economics*, 87: 1298–303.

Roby, J. (2005). Women and children in the global sex trade: Towards a more effective policy. *International Social Work*, 48(2), 136–47.

Sengendo, J. and Nambi, J. (1997). *The Psychological Effect of Orphanhood: A Study of Orphans in Rakai District*. Health Transit Review.

Ssewamala, F.M., Karimli, L., Han, C.K., and Ismayilova, L. (2010). Social capital, savings, and educational performance of orphaned adolescents in Sub-Saharan Africa. *Children and Youth Services Review*, 32, 1704–10.

UNAIDS (2008). *2008 Report on the Global AIDS Epidemic*. Geneva: UNAIDS. www.unaids.org.

UNAIDS (2008a). Report of the UN Secretary General to the General Assembly on the Declaration of Commitment on HIV/AIDS. Geneva: UNAIDS. http://data.unaids.org/pub/report/2008/20080429_sg_progress-report-en.pdf.

UNAIDS (2009). Call for Fully Funded Global Fund to Fight AIDS, Tuberculosis, and Malaria. http://www.unaids.org/en/KnowledgeCentre/Resources/FeatureStories/archive/2009/20090331_GF.asp.

UNAIDS (2010). UNAIDS 2010b Children and AIDS. Fifth Stocktaking Report, 2010. Geneva: UNAIDS.

UNDP (2003). *Evaluation of UNDP's Role in the PRSP Process*. New York: United Nations Development Programme.

UNHCR (2011). African Charter on the Rights and Welfare of the Child. http://www.unhcr.org/refworld/docid/3ae6b38c18.html.

UNICEF (1990). Convention on the Rights of the Child. http://www.unicef-irc.org/portfolios/crc.html#Preamble.

UNICEF (2009). *Progress Report for Children Affected by HIV/AIDS*. New York: UNICEF.

UNICEF (2010). Country statistics: Zimbabwe. http://www.unicef.org/infobycountry/zimbabwe_statistics.html.

UNICEF (2011a). *A Situational Analysis on the Status of Women's and Children's Rights in Zimbabwe, 2005–2010: A Call for Reducing Disparities and Improving Equity*. Harare: UNICEF Zimbabwe.

UNICEF (2011b). *Taking Evidence to Impact: Making a Difference for Vulnerable Children Living in a World with HIV and AIDS*. New York: UNICEF.

UNICEF (2013). Female genital mutilation/cutting. http://www.unicef.org/protection/57929_58002.html.

United Nations (UN) (n.d.). Universal Declaration of Human Rights. http://www.un.org/en/documents/udhr/.

United Nations (UN) (2000). Protocol to Prevent, Suppress and Punish Trafficking in Persons, Especially Women and Children, Supplementing the United Nations Convention Against Transnational Organized Crime. http://www.uncjin.org/Documents/Conventions/dcatoc/final_documents_2/convention_%20traff_eng.pdf.

Walther, T. (2003). Declaration of the rights of the child. http://www.unicef.org/malaysia/1959-Declaration-of-the-Rights-of-the-Child.pdf.

World Health Organization (WHO) (n.d.). Health and Human Rights. http://www.who.int/hhr/Economic_social_cultural.pdf.

Chapter 10

Conclusion: Closing Thoughts

Margaret Lombe, Harriet Mabikke, and Alex Ochumbo

This book set out to develop a comprehensive understanding of the plight of children classified as vulnerable in sub-Saharan Africa. It attempted to bring together in one place data regarding OVC based on a systematic review of literature along with supplemental data drawing upon studies conducted by the authors with children that have been made vulnerable by HIV/AIDS in Kenya and Zambia. The first section of the book highlighted the HIV/AIDS crisis in sub-Saharan Africa and presented an overview of the adult mortality and resultant disproportionate numbers of orphaned children in the region. The book, in the second section, took an in-depth look at the different living arrangements of OVC in Botswana, Kenya, and Zambia. Governmental and community responses to the plight of children in sub-Saharan Africa were highlighted in the third section. Effort was made to situate this conversation within the context of human rights, with specific focus on the rights of the child.

Our goal in writing this book was to provide an overview of existing responses to the phenomenon of OVC. We hope to prompt a reflection and dialogue on the plight of the African child who has been classified as vulnerable. For the authors, this question is a serious moral issue pointing to broad societal malaise. How did the phenomenon of child vulnerability take hold in sub-Saharan Africa? What happened to the familial and extra-familial systems of care that define the spirit of "ubuntu"? How does this experience impact Africa's future? In this book, we have extended an invitation to the reader to grapple with these questions.

This book is also intended to be a platform from which to push African policy-makers, capacity-building and civil society agencies, the African child, the international community and anyone who cares about the welfare of children to provide effective responses to the plight of OVC in sub-Saharan Africa. In essence this is an invitation for the reader to act.

In the closing chapter of this book, we acknowledge that the subject of OVC is highly complex and is rooted in socio-economic, political, and cultural dynamics. We struggle with these dynamics as we try to make sense of the situation of children classified as vulnerable. We recognize the significant effort that has been devoted to understanding this issue. We especially acknowledge the effort of well-intentioned individuals and organizations committed to enhancing the welfare of OVCs.

As we grapple with this subject, we are reminded that the global community has a strong history of rallying together in pursuit of justice, combating diseases and climate challenges. An example in place is the global unity in the fight against polio. Indeed, in the 1980s, the world came together through entities such as the World Health Organization (WHO), Rotary International, the US Centers for Disease Control and Prevention (CDC) and the United Nations Children's Fund (UNICEF) with one goal; to eradicate polio. We are reminded of the slogan "Bye Bye Polio" erupting from every child in Africa. Thanks to efforts such as the Global Polio Eradication Initiative, the world is close to attaining the goal of stamping out polio. We are at a crossroads again! We cannot afford to fail children; the stakes are too high for Africa and the global community! Placing the OVC phenomenon under control may require such an effort. We are hopeful because history is on our side. History is on the side of children classified as vulnerable.

Key Lessons Learned

A number of observations emerged regarding the situation of OVC in sub-Saharan Africa. Notable amongst these is the fact that the number of children classified as vulnerable is growing significantly even though the disease, in many parts of sub-Saharan Africa, has plateaued. Indeed, there are more disease-related mortalities despite the fact that incidences of HIV/AIDS have stabilized. The increase in adult mortality has been explained by the duration of time taken for the pandemic to reach maturity. The observed adult mortality is suggestive; it has not only compromised the welfare of children in the region but also changed the region's landscape. Indeed, classified as OVC are now part of African landscape. The huge numbers of OVC has limited the capacity of familial systems of care, challenging the spirit of ubuntuism. With the fragmentation of ubuntuism, the dignity that traditionally characterized the African child has been compromised. Alongside this is the entry of the NGO culture on the scene, which has allowed traditional systems of care to abdicate their responsibility. The repercussions of this fragmentation will be felt for many years to come unless measures for adequate care of children categorized as vulnerable are put in place.

Another observation made relates to the invisibility and lack of voice for children classified as vulnerable. Indeed, it is common knowledge that a child, in many African communities, is invisible—a non-participant—in the decision-making process at both the family and policy level. This is especially true for young people classified as vulnerable. But if communities OK the "adultified" child, they need to shift the cultural boundaries, enabling participation of children in matters that affect them.

We also learned that, currently, sub-Saharan Africa does not have a comprehensive legal or policy framework for the care and protection of OVCs, leaving a significant proportion of children so classified to slip through the cracks. At the basic level, numerous problems exist. Primary among these is the question of definition. Indeed, the definition of child is highly contested across the region. There are different and oftentimes contradictory definitions of what a child is. Lack of a uniform definition of a child is problematic for policy and programming purposes.

This ambiguity might make children, especially OVCs, more vulnerable and more likely to be negatively impacted in claiming their rights.

Furthermore, the care of children classified as vulnerable continues to be fragmented and uncoordinated. Indeed, anybody can start an OVC related NGO with minimal supervision from both the government and local community. This often leads to duplication of services and has potential for OVC abuse. There is also dearth of programs that focus on rural localities. This may be due to the high overheads associated with working in rural areas. This observation is noteworthy and points to the need for policies aimed at providing guidance to well-meaning agencies serving children characterized as vulnerable. It also challenges policy-makers to put in place mechanisms to encourage capacity-building agencies providing assistance to OVCs to serve rural areas where they may be most needed.

Another factor relates to lack of data assessing program and policy effects on the welfare of OVC. Programs designed for children classified as OVC tend to emphasize magnitude—numbers served—as a yardstick for measuring impact, neglecting other useful indicators in child welfare. This observation is closely connected to the lack of a central database on children classified as vulnerable. In the absence of systematically collected data, policy and program decisions will continue to be made without a sound scientific basis. Additionally, OVC related policy and programming, research has shown, for the most part is externally driven, relying on international organizations. Evidence exists to suggest that, no matter how well-intentioned, internationally driven programming may not be the solution to the OVC problem in Africa, partly due to the high overheads and complexities surrounding the OVC issue. Moreover, in many cases, the children for whom these programs are implemented are not consulted. Children's voices need to be heard in policies related to their wellbeing; they are the primary stakeholders.

Children in our case study, we learned, have a sound understanding of human rights as they relate to children. They also count on adults on whose care they depend to be effective custodians of these rights. Children, in our study, taught us that they have aspirations and understand what they need in order to realize their dreams and aspirations. Indeed, despite the label of "vulnerability," the children desire to be productive members of their communities. One of their needs is quality education, which in fact is a right guaranteed under the CRC.

We also learned how children classified as vulnerable would like to be treated by society—treat them like any other person regardless of their HIV status. There may be a moral lesson in this. This observation pushes us to take pause and reflect on how we relate to each other and to people we consider vulnerable/disadvantaged. The vulnerabilities we see, isms and other labels we use to classify others, often stand in the way of meaningful engagement and interdependence—we all have something to offer! This may also be viewed as a call to rethink labels we use to define children considered vulnerable. Overall, children classified as vulnerable are not different from other young people—they have similar aspirations and dreams. The label "OVC" may need to be evaluated. It is not based on resilience or empowerment models. To the contrary, it is shaped by a deficit narrative that fails to take into consideration the capability and potential of the children so classified.

Policy and Program Recommendations

A number of recommendations flow from the issues examined in this book. We focus narrowly on a few policy and programmatic propositions. With respect to programmatic recommendations, the authors argue that global efforts dedicated to OVC care and wellbeing be channeled through one reputable organization. Indeed, the fragmented efforts currently undertaken by well-meaning individuals, NGOs, and other entities, while laudable, may not be effective in addressing the challenge of OVC in sub-Saharan Africa. The polio eradication initiative presents the global community with a model to draw upon. Globally, effort to tackle the disease was channeled through Rotary Clubs and the World Health Organization; these organizations, in turn, worked directly with health ministries in various countries. This model offered a clear chain of accountability that helped minimize resource wastage and duplication. The American Cancer Society also utilizes a similar model in the fight against cancer.

Recognizing that OVC may be a feature of the African landscape for a long time, we urge communities in Africa to rise to the challenge of taking care of children classified as vulnerable. These communities have the moral authority to take the lead on this issue. Granted, the OVC situation has become a crisis of high proportions but African communities, traditionally, have used their creativity in responding to challenges; traditional coping mechanisms may need to be rediscovered. This call does not negate the important role played by international capacity-building organizations; to the contrary, what it does is to push Africans to take their role of custodianship seriously. Undeniably, the future of sub-Saharan Africa rests on the shoulders of its children, regardless of labels used to classify them.

Furthermore, the authors encourage strengthening community-based systems that support the new reality of child-headed households. Community-based systems of care may involve training of the community members to provide both moral and material support to child-headed households. This support may be a mechanism for the transfer of much needed livelihood sustaining skills and knowledge that children raising other children often lack. Alongside this, we encourage communities to be in the forefront of programs such as meals on wheels to ensure that these children—especially the ones living on the street—are assured of at least one meal per day. The food designated for this program may come from the communities themselves, e.g., a special collection may be held for the education, support, and care of OVC. As the adage goes, "charity begins at home"; before communities look for outside help for support in caring for children made vulnerable, they may have to start from within. The general message in community-based care is that vulnerability amongst children is not acceptable; if each and every one of us plays their part, however small, vulnerability amongst children can be overcome.

At the policy level, we recommend that effort be taken to clearly delineate who a child is. This, as noted earlier, has important implications for the protection of children. Indeed, having a uniform definition of "child" is likely to minimize ambiguity and ensure adequate protection. Alongside this may be efforts directed at raising awareness on the rights of the child and the role of the community in safeguarding these rights. This may also require that mechanisms for follow-through are put in place at the grassroots level to ensure accountability.

In addition, there is need for dialogue between customary and legal law with respect to OVC care and protection, especially around fostering and adoption. While statutory law clearly defines who may adopt or even foster a child, ensuring protection for OVC from potentially unsuitable members of society, this is not extended to immediate, or extended, family members under customary law. Customary law may have provided protection to orphaned children through a mechanism of sanction. This may have worked effectively when the extended family lived in close proximity. This, for the most part, is no longer the case as people tend to migrate to cities and even other countries. In the absence of this protection, upon the death of a parent/s, surviving children may be placed under the care of family members, some of whom may be abusive to the children. Girls may be especially vulnerable. For better protection of OVCs, customary law needs to be closely aligned to other legal frameworks.

Policies that promote gender justice should also be encouraged. Research has shown that in this part of the world, women tend to be better guardians of children. Yet mainly because of their lack of control of productive resources such as land, they are disproportionately represented among the poor, hence the phrase feminization of poverty. For better protection of children, including OVC, focus could be on the implementation of gender-sensitive policies in areas such as land ownership, a sector in which women are grossly under-represented. Alongside this may be enactment of affirmative action type of policies requiring financial institutions to invest meaningfully in women-led ventures. To ensure effectiveness, such policies could include a mechanism of accountability and follow-through at the community level.

Partly because men generally remarry upon the death of a wife, single-father households with respect to OVC tend to be rare. Upon the death of a father, communities in Africa may encourage land and property grabbing by members of the extended family, oftentimes leaving the deceased's wife and children destitute; exposing children to vulnerability. This practice could be penalized. Women and children may need to be educated about their rights in such instances and in other matters pertaining to inheritance.

The authors further recommend that foreign aid be tied to a country's performance in reducing vulnerability among children. This could be implemented in the same manner as the Millennium Development Goals (MDGs). Such a system could establish time-sensitive goals aimed at reducing vulnerability among children. Currently there are no clear guidelines for countries to measure progress or lack of in reducing vulnerability among children. Also, there is no mechanism by which countries may be held responsible for neglecting their responsibilities towards OVC. As with the MDGs, each country could be required to present a performance report to the responsible entity.

To guide policy and program decisions, we recommend development of a central database identifying and recording demographic characteristics of children classified as OVC. These data may need to be aggregated by gender. Data collection could also extend to measuring program effects. Key players in this endeavor may be affected children and their communities.

Appendix A
Questionnaire

Questionnaire # ____ Location ID # ____ Respondent ID # ____

Name of Interviewer ___________ Date of Interview ___/___/___

Orphaned and Vulnerable Children

Hello, my name is ___________. We are writing a book on the plight of children made vulnerable by HIV/AIDS and its correlates. We would like this book to represent the perspective of children. You are one of the children we have selected to learn from. We would like to ask you some questions about yourself, your family, your community and how you are dealing with the dilemma of HIV/AIDS. Your answers to each question are important to us but you can skip any questions you are not comfortable answering. Your answers to all the questions will be confidential. We would like to thank you, in advance, for giving your time and agreeing to participate in this survey. The interview will take about 60 minutes to complete.

Now I'm going to ask you a few questions about yourself and your family.

1. How old are you? ___________
2. What is your gender? Female ____ Male ____
3. Are you currently in school? ____ What is your grade level? ____
4. Have you heard about HIV/AIDS? Can you tell me what you think AIDS is?

   ____

   ____

   ____

5. Do you have AIDS or does anyone you know have AIDS?
   What is the relationship between you and that person?

   ____

   ____

   ____

6. Do you live with your parents or at a home? (institution) _____________
   Can you talk to me about your parents? (are they alive?) _____________
   If no, how did they die and how old were you when they died?

   ____

   ____

   ____

8. Can you tell me how you feel when you think about your parents?

____

____

Why do you think you feel the way you do?

____

____

9. Do your relatives come to visit you? If yes, how do you feel when they visit you? If they do not, how do you feel?

____

____

____

10. If they are alive and you do not live with them, do they come to visit you? If they do, how do they react to you and what do they say to you? How do you relate to them? Can you explain your relationship with them?

____

____

____

11. What would you like them to say to you? Why would you like them to say this?

____

____

____

12. What would you like them to do for you? Why would you like them to do this for you?

____

____

____

Now I want to learn about your life and relationship outside your family or home/institution.

13. Do you currently go to school? If you do, are you happy going to school or do you go because you were asked to go? Please explain your answer.

____

____

____

14. Do you think it is important to go to school? Can you tell me why you think it's important/not important?

____

____

____

15. What are your hopes and goals for the future? What should the institution/ parents do to help you achieve your goals for the future?

16. If you had the power to help, what would you do to help children living with AIDS and those made orphans by AIDS?

Now I am going to ask you a few questions about human rights as they relate to the child.

17. Have you heard of human rights? What does this mean to you?

18. Should children have rights? Should they have the same rights as adults? Please explain your answer.

19. What rights are important to you? Do you enjoy these rights? Please explain your answer.

20. Who is responsible for helping you realize your rights?
    What do you or would you do to ensure you realize your rights?
    If you had power, what would you do to ensure:
    a) children knew about their rights?
    b) realized their rights?
    c) make sure these rights were respected?

Note: Some of the questions (e.g. 21 and 22) in this section only apply to children who are currently living in a home or institution, please skip the questions if need be.

21. If you are currently living in a home/institution, can you tell me about your life at the home/institution?
Are you happy at the institution?
If yes, explain why you are happy. If not, why not?
How long have you lived in the home/institution?

____
____
____

22. If you are currently living in a home/institution, if you had power to change things, what would you change to improve the lives of children at your home/institution?

____
____
____

23. How are you treated by others (children and adults)?
Why do you think you are treated this way?

____
____
____

24. How would you like to be treated by others?
Why would you like to be treated this way?

____
____
____

Index

Bold page numbers indicate figures, *italic* numbers indicate tables.